GRAND CENTRAL

LARGE PRINT

Also by Kevin Hazzard

American Sirens

The Incredible Story of the Black Men Who Became America's First Paramedics

A Thousand Naked Strangers

A Paramedic's Wild Ride to the Edge and Back

NO ONE'S COMING

THE ROGUE HEROES OUR GOVERNMENT TURNS TO WHEN THERE'S NOWHERE ELSE TO TURN

KEVIN HAZZARD

GCP
GRAND CENTRAL
LARGE PRINT

Grand Central Publishing
Hachette Book Group
1290 Avenue of the Americas, New York, NY 10104
grandcentralpublishing.com
@grandcentralpub

First Edition: March 2026

Grand Central Publishing is a division of Hachette Book Group, Inc. The Grand Central Publishing name and logo is a registered trademark of Hachette Book Group, Inc.

Print book interior design by Bart Dawson.

Library of Congress Control Number: 2025948356

ISBNs: 978-0-306-83518-6 (hardcover), 978-0-306-83520-9 (ebook), 978-1-538-78317-7 (large print)

For Jay and Vika

And all the people fighting to make the world they'll inherit a better place

CONTENTS

No one is coming. It's up to us.

—motto, Phoenix Air medical team

The king called up his jet fighters, he
said you better earn your pay

—The Clash

NO ONE'S COMING

PART ONE

1

CARTERSVILLE, GEORGIA
PRESENT DAY

Morning in North Georgia, and the massive steel doors of an unmarked hangar slowly roll open to reveal what looks at first like a shipping container. It's forty-four feet long, eight feet wide, and painted the obscene white of a sterile field. It was conceived by the State Department, designed by Big Tech, tested by national security contractors, privately funded, and flown here by the Air Force. The US government loves an acronym and they named it the CBCS, or Containerized Biocontainment System, but really what you're looking at is a way to bring people home when they're far away and dying of something horrible. SARS, malaria, tuberculosis. All the hemorrhagic fevers. The container is here in this hangar because what existed before was ingenious but too small—it couldn't scale up to match the pace of deadly pathogens. A healthy fear of those pathogens is the angel in the container's architecture. It is one container among several and by itself has the capacity to hold four critically ill and highly contagious patients, plus their doctors, and was meant to be transported two abreast inside a 747, an aircraft so big it can swallow six of them with room left over. The CBCS was so far ahead of its time when it was introduced in 2015 that if six containers had been loaded onto a 747 that one aircraft would've represented more infectious disease bed space than existed in all US hospitals combined. Force multiplier may not be a strong enough term. This container and the others like it serve as testament to both our present preparedness and also to our past failures—at once hope and wrath. Because implicit in any rescue is the unavoidable fact that the worst has already occurred.

2

BEECH MOUNTAIN, NORTH CAROLINA
JULY 2014

Dent Thompson stepped out into the rolling splendor of an Appalachian afternoon. It was Friday and he'd been on vacation since Sunday. The week had started with plumbing issues, nothing trivial. The entire basement had flooded, but that was behind him now, or mostly behind him, and Dent had finally settled into the languid rhythm of a long vacation. He had a Bud Light and a magazine, eased himself into a deck chair, and took a deep breath. Dent's parents built this place. His dad designed it to look like a Swiss chalet with a gabled roof and exposed beams, that ornately carved molding. It sat on a piece of land 4,500 feet up the side of Beech Mountain in North Carolina, and after they were gone, they left it to Dent. From this spot he could look for a hundred miles over the vast woodland of the Tennessee Divide. Since inheriting the house, Dent and his wife, Pepper, regularly made the five-hour drive north from Atlanta. They had a close group of friends on the mountain, and before dinner they'd all sit on the porch and forget anyplace else existed.

Dent took a long sip of beer. His life in Atlanta was hectic beyond measure but here there was nothing except the denim blue of a summer sky, no sound at all but the birds or maybe Pepper—Southern, opinionated, never at rest—inside the house and raising a minor ruckus. He'd just opened his magazine when his cell rang. The screen showed a 202 area code.

Washington, DC.

He answered on the first ring.

"Dent, it's Walters from State. Would that system you have work for Ebola?"

It was 3 p.m. on Friday, July 25.

Dent didn't know Walters. Not really. He knew his full name was William Walters, that he was an Army veteran and a doctor who now ran an obscure organization within the State Department called Operational Medicine, which sounded to Dent like something out of a spy novel. The two had met a few months earlier during the Winter Olympics in Sochi. Dent and his brother, Mark, own a Georgia-based company called Phoenix Air, and during the Games they had a contract to shuttle presidential envoys to Russia and run medical standby for visiting Americans. Should've been routine, but Vladimir Putin was denying visas and barring entry and overall making life difficult for foreign businesses and governments and Dent and Walters had briefly teamed up for what at the time seemed like a major issue but which now, suddenly, (had Walters really said Ebola?) felt like it'd never been a problem at all.

Whatever ease Dent felt just a moment ago was gone. He shifted in his deck chair.

"For what now?"

"That biocontainment capability you talked about," Walters said. "I need to know if it works."

A pause. "Yeah, it works."

Walters already knew Dent would say yes—salesmen sell and Dent's a world-class salesman. Right away he shot back: "No, for real. Because the next thing that comes out of my mouth is me saying that you have to use it."

That's how fast it happened. A warm afternoon, nothing but tranquility, and then the United States government—the most powerful force on Earth—was calling him for help. Imagine God extending a finger across the cracked ceiling of the Sistine Chapel. Dent swallowed hard. Here things started moving fast. Walters is almost shockingly direct and told Dent without preamble that a couple of Americans were dying of Ebola in Africa (exact number and location unknown) and that no one else on Earth (literally, they'd tried) would or even could get them home. So more or less their only hope was Phoenix Air.

About that time Dent felt the bottom drop out. This was supposed to be a vacation but here he was, the beer slowly going warm in his hand, getting pulled into the deep end of something big. All Dent knew about Ebola was what everyone knew about Ebola—that it's deadly and contagious and absolutely horrifying. That you liquify from the inside and then watch as the life drips out of you. That there's no cure. His mind went to biblical plagues, to panic in the streets, to dying the most horrible death imaginable. To fear. Paralyzing fear. He thought about his employees and whether he could convince them to take this chance and if he even wanted to. Unsaid here but certainly not overlooked was the question of whether they *should* bring Ebola to the American continent. Seemed like inviting the unthinkable. There was also the very real fact that he didn't know the first thing about Ebola or how to safely transport people who had it. He didn't even know how many people they were talking about or where they were or what hospital would consider taking such a patient. He *did* know that the risks were huge, almost incalculable, and he knew too that nobody would blame him for saying no. Phoenix didn't have to do this.

And yet.

Call it bravery or confidence, maybe overconfidence, a cowboy mentality—whatever the word for it is—but for over two decades Phoenix Air had been making its name by saying yes when everybody else said no. But first he had questions. The system Walters had called about was a highly advanced but wholly unproven piece of technology that Phoenix had created to fit inside the passenger compartment of a Gulfstream III aircraft. It was basically a one-person negative pressure tent, capable (in theory) of keeping even the most dangerous pathogens from getting out. The CDC had run it through an extensive proving process and certified that it had the ability to contain just about every known virus *except* Ebola. And though it had been thoroughly tested, it'd never been used. This was not an insignificant detail—a twelve-hour Atlantic crossing is no place to learn your experimental technology turns into a pumpkin at hour six.

"We don't know anything about Ebola," he told Walters. "But if you can bring down the government's top doctors to tell me this thing is safe, we'll do it."

Walters said, "I'll call you right back."

A click. Then nothing. In the silence, Dent's anxiety began to recede. He was once again on vacation, sitting on his deck with nothing but the green blanket of trees visible from his perch on Beech Mountain.

The conversation he just had couldn't exist here. Too quiet, too peaceful. And anyway, his demand that the government send its medical experts to inspect his technology—they'd never agree to that. Walters would call someone else. There'd be no more talk of Ebola. He leaned back, drank his beer. The trees pressed in. The world faded. He relaxed. He forgot. Then his cell rang.

The 202 area code again.

3

Dent Thompson's probably about the last person you'd expect to find in this situation. He looks like the sort of moderately successful guy who's recently retired and now plays golf and gets dragged by his wife to parties. And maybe he would be if it not for his younger brother, Mark, because it was Mark Thompson who parlayed a short stint in the military and a love for skydiving into one of the most peculiar companies in America. Mark in both person and legend is unmistakably a pilot. He's self-assured and laconic, the embodiment of Chuck Yeager, with thinning, windswept brown hair and a mouth forever curled into a faint smile like someone's told him a joke he can't share. He was born and raised in Atlanta and when he talks, if you close your eyes, it's Billy Bob Thornton you hear. He's been at the controls, variously, of an airplane or a helicopter or a race car since Richard Nixon was president. His misadventures, too numerous to count, include almost buying an airplane from suspected drug runners, going airborne and nearly dying after flipping a race car in Daytona, and briefly getting detained by US Customs agents while returning to the United States carrying Muammar Gaddafi's suitcase nuke. Mark Thompson does not rattle easily.

And whatever Mark is, Dent by nearly every significant metric is his opposite. Dent is shorter and, despite an in-house personal trainer, rounder. He's been described as looking like a painting of the fifth earl of somewhere, with wispy white hair and matching eyebrows that dance across his forehead and soften his imperious demeanor. Dent has a way of becoming the center of every conversation. Always talking, always selling, the kind of guy who works even the smallest problem from two or three different angles. You want him on your side. Where Mark is unflappable, Dent exists in a constant state of flap. It's what keeps him vigilant, what's made him so wildly successful. Decades at Phoenix have not left him immune to the romance of their work and, as often happens, when Dent reaches the point where a weird story gets weirder—like the time he bought an airplane from the Saudis while standing on an island in North Georgia wearing nothing but a bathing suit—his quick but measured voice pirouettes into high-pitched peels of excitement. Mark's voice, when he talks, is so soft you have to lean in to hear it.

Their divergent personalities are deeply embedded in the company's DNA. In describing Phoenix, one pilot's wife shook her head and said simply, "Assembly of characters, my friend. Assembly of characters." It's an eccentric place and those eccentricities are byproducts of the radically different but reluctantly inextricable Thompson brothers. And so are its successes. In fact, if either of them ever stopped long enough to consider what had brought him to this particular witch's house—how, after Ebola hit, Phoenix became the only outfit on Earth our government could turn to—each would find that the trail of breadcrumbs led straight back to his own brother.

*

By the time Dent Thompson was eligible to be drafted into Vietnam the government had instituted a lottery system. It's hard to imagine now but at the beginning of each year a television station would broadcast the drawing of draft numbers. Picture a big spinning bingo basket with a man from the Rotary Club turning the handle. Inside were balls numbered from 1 through 365. For each day of the year, a numbered ball would be drawn and that would be the draft number assigned to it. Low numbers got drafted first and anything over 100 was basically an exemption. In 1968, Dent turned eighteen and became draft eligible. His birthday is March 23, and the bingo ball for that date was 240. Dent was exempted.

In an instant the threat of Vietnam was behind him, leaving Dent with an open but uncertain future. He went to college and decided afterward, of all places, to work at Disney World. When Walt opened his new amusement park in October 1971, Orlando was just a malarial outpost in the central Florida wasteland. Nothing but orange groves and dirt roads, more cattle than hotels. Dent arrived a few months later, along with thousands of recent college grads from all over the globe who wanted to be part of Disney World's first summer. He got hired as a boat captain for the Jungle Cruise and partied all night with a batch of twentysomethings whose first taste of the real world was employee housing at the happiest place on Earth. It was the wildest time of his life. He decided to stay, got married (then divorced), and watched Orlando grow. And all the while Dent was working the angles. As a former communications major, he got talked into writing newsletters for the various employee clubs established to keep Disney's young and rambunctious workforce out of trouble. The work was unpaid and even less glamorous, but Dent took it seriously.

To anyone else, this would've been a burden, something done for a favor or a six pack, but Dent saw it as a way to distinguish himself. His newsletters went to everyone on their respective distribution lists, and here Dent sensed an opportunity. To each list of recipients, along with the names of active members in good standing, Dent added the people above them—way above them. Department heads and regional directors, vice presidents, presidents, basically everyone short of Walt Disney himself stared in utter confusion once a month at the latest dispatch from the Scuba Club. It was a lot of extra work but Dent kept at it and pretty soon upper management took notice and he was rescued from the Jungle Cruise and brought into corporate communications where, in short order, he was placed in charge. And he stayed there, in Orlando, at Disney, perfectly content. Until a decade later, when he wasn't.

As Dent headed home for the 1983 Christmas holiday, he was ready for a new start. And if the life he'd so far built for himself was coming to an end, then Mark's was just beginning.

It had occurred to Mark Thompson, as he walked into the Army recruitment office and saw a poster of a helicopter hanging on the wall, that it'd be better to fly than walk and so he decided on the spot to be a pilot. It was 1969 and unlike Dent, Mark's July 9 birthday was assigned draft number 1. He was going to Vietnam. Rather than waiting for his conscription date, he enlisted, was given his pick of jobs, and chose flying. By the time he finished basic and then flight school, the war was winding down and fewer soldiers were being shipped to Vietnam. He was offered an early release and took it. There wasn't much need in the civilian world for well-trained but inexperienced helicopter pilots, so he got fixed wing certified and started flying small planes. Not because he loved to fly but because he loved to skydive. The logic here is tricky to follow, but in a classic example of the risk-equals-reward Thompson ethos, Mark figured there'd be more opportunities to jump from planes if he was also the one flying them. Mark by then was back in school and out of money and somehow managed to convince the dean of his small university to add skydiving to the curriculum as an elective—with Mark as instructor, chief pilot, and occasional participant.

Over time his recreational skydiving led to educational skydiving, which birthed a skydiving business, which gradually morphed into an air freight business that Mark quickly lost to his partners in a hostile takeover. And it was from the ashes of that failed venture that a new company arose.

Sort of.

Mark's an entrepreneur and ideas guy, but like big picture thinkers everywhere he lacks the focus to sew up the details and see projects all the way to fruition. For that reason—along with a not inconsequential lack of cash flow—by the winter of 1983 Mark's second air freight business, which he named Phoenix Air, had stalled. He needed help. At least, that's what Dent had come all the way up from Orlando to tell him. Dent was done with Disney and wanted to return permanently to Atlanta, to join forces with Mark and turn this struggling one-man business into a family-run juggernaut. Mark wasn't sure he needed a partner, but he knew his brother had the patience and salesmanship, the vast reserves of nervous energy to throw at the logistical and regulatory hurdles that lay between the floundering Phoenix Air and long-term success. Mark said yes and Dent packed the remains of his Orlando life onto a moving truck and came home.

It wasn't long before Dent figured out why Phoenix was flatlining. For starters, the company's headquarters sat in Mark's basement and consisted of nothing but a lone desk and matching credenza, both overflowing with paperwork. Every communication Mark had gotten from the FAA about regulations and the corresponding proof that Phoenix was, in fact, in compliance—literally thousands of documents—was stuffed into drawers with no organization at all. Dent commandeered the files and got the company's affairs in order, and it's here that another, even more troubling, picture began to emerge. Phoenix specialized in flying automotive parts to assembly plants around the country, but there were a million companies who specialized in flying automotive parts to assembly plants around the country. There was so much competition that none of them, Phoenix included, were making any money. Dent figured they had two options—either continue on and risk being driven out of business by an overcrowded marketplace or strike out in a new direction entirely. Salvation required a big idea, so their first fork-in-the-road moment was also a chance for Mark to stake his claim as resident visionary. As it turned out, he did have an idea, a big one, an idea he was certain couldn't fail. Dent sat up in his chair. Mark leaned back.

"We're gonna start flying explosives."

Cue the cymbal clash. You can almost see Dent's mouth flopping open as Mark paced the room, explaining how only two companies were licensed to fly explosives in US airspace and how both of them, according to their pilots, were breaking the law. Mark knew the pilots and they'd told him that despite FAA regulations strictly forbidding it, planes loaded with dynamite were routinely left sitting unattended on crowded runways. In cities all over America. Sometimes overnight. It was only a matter of time before federal regulators caught on and shut them down, and once that happened there'd be no competition because there just aren't that many pilots willing to strap themselves into an aircraft full of dynamite. But it was Mark's kind of crazy. Hell, he told Dent, the only reason he hadn't done it already was the long and tedious approval process, but then that's exactly what his brother had signed on to handle.

"So. Are you in or not?"

Scrapping your entire business model and wading through miles of red tape and countless bureaucratic cul-de-sacs just to come out on the other side as one of a handful of companies willing to risk blowing itself up over the American Midwest isn't most people's idea of an attractive offer. You could've forgiven Dent for saying no. But there's this other, unexpected, wrinkle to Dent's personality, possibly the lone attribute the brothers share—Dent Thompson can't stand to be bored.

Going all the way back to college when he picked up overnight shifts on an ambulance just for fun, Dent has always sought out adventure. While working for Disney, first as captain of the Jungle Cruise and later in corporate communications, he got restless and applied to be a reserve officer with the Orange County Sheriff's

Office. He worked in uniform patrol and the narcotics division. Mostly at night, always alone. Late one night he was dispatched to a little community south of Orlando called Taft where someone was driving around shooting into houses. It was quiet and dark when he arrived. Dent pulled over at the intersection of two dirt roads to listen for gunshots and saw a pair of taillights about a hundred yards off. He had just stepped from his cruiser to stare into the distance when he saw a muzzle flash, followed immediately by the crack of a bullet hitting the telephone pole just above his head and then the report of a large caliber rifle. *Flash, smack, BOOM.* Death had missed him by inches.

Dent dove into a drainage ditch and looked up just in time to see the car headed right for him. Call it an answered prayer but the car sped by and kept on going. Dent jumped in his cruiser and fell in behind the speeding car, yelling into the radio that he'd been shot at and was now in pursuit. Both cars raced along in a hail of dust and kicked up rocks until the road ended abruptly at a stand of cypress trees. The suspects stopped. Dent stopped. He flipped on his spotlight, flung open his door to crouch behind it and then thrust his pistol through the open driver's side window. He was yelling into the PA—"Stay where you are, keep your hands where I can see 'em!"—when the department's helicopter arrived and cast the whole thing into chaos. The rotor wash stirred up a tornado of dirt and debris and drowned out all sound. Dent had no idea where the suspects were or what they were doing. He was screaming for the helicopter to back off when in his left ear he caught the unmistakable sound of someone racking a shotgun shell. *CH-CH.* The neurology of fear and survival collided in a terrifying instant, and it all became clear. A shooter had disappeared in the rotor wash, crept around behind him, and this was it. He was dead. But the shot never came. Dent peeked over his shoulder and there, crouching next to him, wasn't a killer but another sheriff's deputy, who had arrived unnoticed in all the madness. Dent was jangly from the chemical response to near-death (twice over) but he was still alive. With a lazy Florida moon hanging over the pines, he arrested, booked, and jailed the shooters, then disappeared into the night to resume patrol.

This was the guy Mark had brought on to serve as counterpoint to his own cowboy flamboyance. To be the sober voice of reason. And so, yeah. Phoenix Air started flying explosives.

4

The process for obtaining the clearance to fly explosives in civilian aircraft through US airspace, taking off and landing in cities across the country, quite literally a ticking timebomb, is every bit as long and tortured as it sounds. But Dent proved true to his word and saw it through. He filed and refiled the papers, submitted forms in triplicate, organized site visits, and underwent interviews. He endured. And after two years Phoenix abandoned auto parts for dynamite and blasting caps. Now that they'd slipped through the door, the brothers—who just a few months before were borrowing money for jet fuel—took it even further. They decided to specialize in only the most dangerous, difficult jobs and after another two-year process, became licensed to carry *high* explosives. They flew all over the world, to Norway and Indonesia, Malaysia, Australia, Afghanistan, everywhere, delivering down-well charges for the oil industry, and ejector seats, bombs, missiles, and rockets for the US military. They were now way out over the edge, and by the mid-80s, Mark had flown everywhere but Antarctica with the most dangerous cargo imaginable.

They'd gotten so busy Mark couldn't do it all himself. It was time to hire pilots, but this was no ordinary casting call. They needed reliable, capable pilots, sure, but those skills can be learned. Mark insists he could teach a monkey to land a jet. The need for adventure, however, is either there or it's not. And if it's not, if a pilot would be happy just to shuttle passengers from Dayton to Chicago and back, then however good he might be, he'd not likely say yes when asked to fly into the Horn of Africa during a shooting war. For that they needed people comfortable operating in and around danger, people who meticulously and unfailingly follow every single regulation every single time, who are okay with lots of travel and no personal space, people who take the job seriously but also—because it can be so incredibly serious—are capable of laughing at it all. The right pilots would contain that delicate balance of sacred and profane. Though it wouldn't happen until later, when Phoenix was much more established and had expanded into medical flights, few stories represent the gonzo lore of Phoenix Air and its people better than the Anchorage Beer Run.

Picture two bored pilots on a days-long layover. They're sitting around the FBO, fixed-base operator, at the Anchorage airport waiting for a jet inbound from Asia. Major airports typically have an FBO that handles the smaller jets like the kind Phoenix flies. And Phoenix pilots are here so often—Anchorage is generally how they reenter the US when coming in off the Pacific—that they have the run of the place. They even keep a car there. An SUV. Bright yellow. These two pilots are sitting around the FBO with nothing but free time and a car, and they decide to make a beer run. Alaskan Amber had become almost fabled at Phoenix, and this was the only place you could get it. So if you're flying through Anchorage, you grab some. And etiquette says if you're getting some for yourself, then you get some for everybody else too.

The pilots buy beer for themselves, plus a case each for the incoming flight crew and, well, there's the medical team on board, and the guys back home who like it, and oh yeah, they'll be landing in Washington and wouldn't it be a nice gesture to get a case for the ambassador. Pretty soon the SUV is full of Alaskan Amber. They slam the tailgate shut and head back to the FBO. And here's where the two worlds of Phoenix Air meet. The first plane took off from an undisclosed location, part of a secret and incredibly delicate mission into an unfriendly country where an American citizen had been held hostage and brutalized and now, after months of negotiations through intermediary nations, has finally been released. His condition is fragile and there are questions about whether or not he'll survive the long international flight. The plan is for the jet to touch down in Anchorage where the first crew will get out of the cockpit and the second will jump in and fly home. Easy.

Except somehow the media has gotten wind of the flight and their secret mission is no longer a secret. Dent's found out about this and calls up the pilots to say reporters will be there, so keep a low profile. Absolutely reasonable advice, but he's telling them this as they're pulling up to the FBO in a bright yellow SUV packed full of pilots and beer. This kicks off a quick discussion—you can't be seen loading beer onto a plane like *Smokey and the Bandit*, but then you can't just leave it on the tarmac either. So a pilot jumps out of the truck, runs into the FBO, and grabs a box of trash bags. Back in Cartersville watching the news, Dent sees his airplane, the one carrying a freed hostage, being loaded with a dozen or more boxes wrapped in black plastic labeled *medical supplies*. The newscasters discussing these mystery supplies either don't notice or fail to mention the condensation beading up on the packaging.

So gradually Mark found his pirates. Some he recruited himself, some heard about Phoenix through stories told in barrooms all across the world and showed up in Cartersville on the off chance they were true. They arrived just in time. Reagan's government was focused on the Soviet Union, on Berlin and Nicaragua and Beirut. Nobody paid much attention to what was being flown where. Things got pretty wild. One night on an island off the west coast of Africa two Phoenix pilots touched down with a load of down-well charges for a remote drilling site. A group of terrified executives ran out on the tarmac screaming that they couldn't accept the delivery, that while the plane was in the air a coup had broken out and if they were caught accepting explosives they'd be treated as participants. But the pilots couldn't return home with the explosives, and after a tense negotiation on the runway, the executives loaded them all into the trunk of a Cadillac so they could be carted off and hidden. The pilots lifted off as the Cadillac sped away and rebels closed in on the airfield.

It might've gone on like this forever if not for the drug-using, womanizing Texas congressman Charlie Wilson, whose obsession with fighting communism led to a massive, and more or less unregulated, covert weapons program. For a decade, the US had been funneling hundreds of millions of dollars in weaponry to help the Afghan mujahideen defeat the Soviet Union. It was Wilson's pet project and when it finally paid off, and the Russians limped home, those weapons were (perhaps not surprisingly) pointed at the West. A chastened American government now wanted accountability. Anyone moving explosives around US airspace was subject to renewed scrutiny. Certifications were no longer enough. Entire facilities needed security clearances and so did anyone working at a cleared facility—from pilots on down to the guy sweeping the floor. Many other companies simply walked away, but Dent threw himself into the additional screening and when they emerged, Phoenix, though still a tiny operation, found itself at the top of the hazardous cargo pyramid. The calls came flooding in.

Becoming the company that'll do anything, no matter how crazy, leads to strange places, but in the case of Phoenix at least, the path was rooted in personality. Mark is guided less by corporate strategy than the desire to have fun, and Dent follows an always-be-closing sales credo, and when put together these complementary philosophies elegantly sum up the Phoenix ethos: Never say no. So even as the requests got wilder, Dent would respond by saying, "Of course we can do that." Then he'd hang up and start yelling, "Now how in hell are we gonna do that?" The logic of figuring out how to pull off the impossible only after agreeing to do it—like becoming a pilot just so you can jump out of planes—is convoluted but born of necessity. Survival among aeronautical giants and entrenched government contractors, among prickly federal bureaucracies, took nerve and expertise but also flexibility. That in many ways Phoenix remained a company in miniature only helped. The legal team responsible for vetting these dangerous and complex missions was a single lawyer; upper-level management—the brain trust tasked with developing creative interpretations that stretched, without violating, FAA regulations—would fit into a single compact car. The mandate was clear, the chain of command simple. Dent could freely say yes to everything. So he did.

For most of the 1990s Phoenix managed Midway Island for the US government, overseeing the Pacific atoll's growing ecotourism industry; in the Caribbean they flew planes retrofitted with radio and television equipment out of a base in Key West, broadcasting sports and international news to the Cuban people as part of a State Department effort, code-named Radio Martí, to undermine Fidel Castro. In the immediate run-up to Operation Desert Storm in 1990, Phoenix flew eighty-three Patriot missile warheads out of Dover Air Force Base, slipped into an informal, multinational backchannel that included a high-level Dutch government official named Hans van der Maat, and ultimately helped deliver the missiles to Saudi Arabia.

That mission was done so quickly and quietly that the only piece of paper on the entire operation was a letter Dent wrung from the Department of Defense, which served as a Get Out of Jail Free card in case some over-eager border agent pegged the pilots for terrorists and had them detained. In 2001, after anthrax-laced letters killed five Americans across four states, the CDC began stockpiling vaccines for any virus likely to be weaponized. The one thing they didn't have was smallpox, so the US reached out to the only person who did—Vladimir Putin. The two governments worked out a deal and Phoenix was sent across the Atlantic and back to deliver vials of Russian smallpox to the US. Each success only further solidified their reputation as discreet practitioners of strange missions. And at the opaque convergence of foreign relations and international commerce there's no shortage of strange.

It was late on a spring afternoon in April 2004 when the call came in. Department of Energy was on the phone explaining to Dent how Libyan dictator and global provocateur Muammar Gaddafi feared the US wanted him dead (he was right) and had reached out to the American government to see about getting himself straight with the West. What followed was a complicated process involving protracted negotiations between three sovereign states that had been dragging on since the Clinton administration but now, finally, only one concession remained—for Gaddafi to turn over his nuclear weapons. Experts were already disassembling them but someone needed to fly the radioactive fissile material back to the US for storage at a government nuclear facility in Alamogordo, New Mexico. Phoenix Air was the first name—possibly the only name—on the DOE's short list and so, the man on the phone asked, would they be willing to do it. There was silence on Dent's end of the line.

"Hello?"

"I'm listening," Dent said.

The caller started talking faster now, assuring Dent that the Department of Energy would provide a stainless steel canister to store the nuclear material, plus a second just in case the first leaked(!). They also threw in an expert from the Oak Ridge National Laboratory in Tennessee. Aside from an aircraft, all that was required of Phoenix was to find a pilot willing to spend twelve hours in close quarters with a recently unspooled nuclear weapon. Dent put his hand over the receiver and yelled to Mark, whose office was only a wall away. Mark stepped out and leaned against the door—one leg crossed over the other, like an old ax handle. He had a cup of coffee in his hand and a pilot's shirt with epaulets tucked into faded jeans. His big silver belt buckle, worn smooth over the years, shined in the overhead light.

Dent nodded his head at the phone: "DOE. They wanna know if we'll go to Libya and pick up Gaddafi's nuclear bombs."

Mark sipped his coffee. "Yeah, I think I'd like to fly that one."

Phoenix's maintenance department removed the passenger seats of a Learjet 36 business-class airplane so the stainless steel drum provided by the Department of Energy to hold the confiscated fissile material could be secured (way) in the back of the aircraft. Mark and his copilot, Mike Ott, took off from Cartersville and flew to Oak Ridge National Laboratory to pick up Stan Moses, the government's leading expert on nuclear weapons. From there they headed east to Tripoli, where Moses was whisked off to a cave in the Libyan mountains where the weapons had been stored. Mark and Mike hit the town. A government handler showed them around the capitol and the Roman ruins and even let them pose for pictures in the dictator's throne room. After two days word came that everything was ready. The pilots returned to their aircraft and once the stainless steel container was loaded, Mark fired up the engines and lifted off into the North African sky. Libya was no longer a nuclear-armed nation.

Getting to this point had taken six years, two American presidents, and an untold number of diplomats. Over the preceding two weeks alone there'd been phone calls for clearances and permissions, for advice, for the notification of every relevant official on the Eastern Seaboard. All this before the plane could blast off for Libya and yet somehow, despite all this planning, no one had bothered to notify the nightwatchman in Bangor.

It was 2 a.m. in Maine when the lone US Customs agent working the graveyard shift at Bangor International Airport heard the first click of his Geiger counter. He carried two—one mounted to the front of his SUV and a second dangling from his belt, both set to detect the long-range alpha waves commonly emitted from smuggled nuclear material. They went off in unison. Beyond the customs building, Bangor International was quiet. But the clicking continued, then sped up, then became constant. A metronome keeping time to the rhythm of apocalypse. Whatever was billowing radiation into the night sky was getting closer. The agent stepped outside, turned toward the vast darkness of the Atlantic, and wondered what horrible thing was coming his way.

Mark was six miles out and closing fast. The Learjet roared in off the ocean, slowed for final approach, then gently touched down and taxied straight to the customs ramp. Mark pulled to a stop and powered down the engines. He opened the door directly behind the left seat, lowered the two-step ladder and was met by a flashlight beam and a customs agent who everyone would later agree was absolutely freaking the fuck out. It took a second to process, but Mark heard the mad click of the Geiger counter first and then, over it, the agent screaming:

"GET AWAY FROM THE AIRPLANE!"

Mark hooked his thumbs beneath his belt buckle, staring with mild fascination at the agent who by now was levitating with white hot anger. He stepped down onto the tarmac. The agent, who refused to get closer than fifty feet, demanded to know what in hell they'd brought into the US that'd set off Geiger counters from six miles out. Mark prefaced what he was about to say with assurances that all of this had been authorized by the sort of important people who authorize these kinds of things. *So, remember, it's okay.* Then, casually, he explained that there was a nuclear bomb on the plane. Or parts of one anyway. Depleted uranium or enriched uranium maybe. Whatever kind could be weaponized, that's what he had. If this response was meant to ease the tension, it did not work.

The agent flung his arms out in a mix of fear and impotent rage: "You've contaminated the whole country!"

At this point Stan Moses stepped forward. It was

the Geiger counter that'd kicked this hornet's nest in the first place, so he approached the agent and held out his hand. "Let me see that thing."

The agent was so thrown by their sudden, radioactive arrival that he actually unclipped the device from his belt and handed it over. Moses, a trained engineer and expert at the government's top nuclear research facility, is also a plainspoken son of Appalachia. After turning the Geiger counter over in his hand, he tossed it back to the agent. He'd figured out the problem: "This thing here's a piece of shit."

Maybe there had been a moment where the situation could've deescalated, where this whole thing might've been okay. That moment was now over.

"Give me your IDs! You're coming with me!"

A phone rang 650 miles south in DC. The head of US Customs and Border Protection's nuclear bureau, woken from a deep sleep, lifted the receiver and caught a panicked torrent of questions and expletives. Something about radiation and Geiger counters and nuclear weapons. This story has become legend and so there are differing versions of what happened next. One version has Stan Moses getting on the phone to explain to the bureau chief who he is and what he's doing, then handing the phone back and listening quietly as the agent gets reamed out. In another, the bureau chief interrupts the agent to ask if he has in his office a copy of the manual on the importation and safe handling of radioactive material.

The agent nods at the phone. "Yes."

"Get it down," the bureau chief says.

The agent grabs the manual off a shelf and drops it on his desk.

"You see the author's name on the cover?"

The agent nods. "Yeah."

"Read it to me."

"Stan Moses."

A pause over the line. Then: "That man sitting across from you? *He's* Stan Moses."

Then the line goes dead.

After that they were free to go. Another crew flew the airplane the final leg of its journey to Alamogordo. Mark went home and told the whole thing to Dent, and over time it became just another in a long line of stories you simply couldn't make up.

5

Phoenix's shift into the air medical world started slowly. They didn't even have medical people on staff, just flew other people's doctors around. Some domestic air ambulance company would get a request to repatriate an American injured on a North Sea oil rig or a sick tourist in Sri Lanka and knowing Phoenix already went to those places, they'd call Dent to see if he could supply an aircraft. The company did enough of these in the early 2000s for the medevac business to hit their radar as an opportunity. To create a medevac division Mark and Dent tapped Bob Tracey, a man who even by Phoenix Air's "assembly of characters" standard, tends to stand out. Bob is something of a marketing savant. He started his career at the Philip Morris tobacco company, was assigned to the Virginia Slims Tour where he worked with tennis great Billie Jean King as she dragged women's tennis into the modern era, and later helped cement and grow Marlboro's sponsorship of the European Formula 1 racing circuit.

He was doing contract work for Philip Morris in 1989 when the Soviet Union collapsed and was asked to slip through the rapidly deteriorating Iron Curtain to work out a cigarette distribution deal. He arrived in Russia to find a country in chaos. Bob wasn't there long before one of his counterparts at another tobacco company was murdered in a contract negotiation gone wrong. He hopped the next train out and soon after landed at Phoenix.

Bob had no experience with the air medical business prior to creating one within Phoenix, so he started meeting with industry experts and soon learned what the Thompson brothers had already suspected—just as there was a need to rush explosives *into* far flung places, there was also a constant need to rush sick and injured people *out* of them. He figured out how much money and what equipment he'd need to get his division off the ground and acquired both, but staffing was a trickier issue. Doctors were reluctant to give up their comfortable jobs and enviable schedules to spend eighteen cramped hours providing critical care in the back of a small aircraft. He hung up flyers in every hospital in the area but got no bites. Then one day Mike Flueckiger walked through the door.

Flueckiger, who'd eventually become known at Phoenix simply as Dr. Mike, was in his 50s. He has floppy hair and a soft voice, and grew up in a large

Mennonite family, one of six Flueckiger kids in a Midwestern town of a couple thousand. He was the first person in his family to go to college, became an ER doctor, and moved to Atlanta to follow his wife's career. He's a gentle soul who rides his bicycle for hours around Atlanta to decompress, who is entirely and disarmingly self-assured, and when he shakes your hand, there's a warmth, an openness, a sort of loose-limbed bearing that calls to mind Kermit the Frog. Which makes this other side of Dr. Mike tough to square. He's a risk-taker, an adventurer, a guy who in 1994 started working for International SOS, a medevac insurance company that for life and death scenarios keeps a small stable of doctors on staff and ready to deploy around the world. For a decade Dr. Mike flew part-time with SOS—to the mountains, the jungle, to rural Mongolia—until he heard about Phoenix Air. So he stopped in for a visit.

Bob Tracey offered him the role of medical director on the spot.

Phoenix being Phoenix, they made their mark with a willingness to transport any type of patient. When an American diagnosed with a highly infectious disease violated a court-ordered quarantine and bounced around Europe before he was caught and placed in federal custody, it was Phoenix who flew him home. Their characteristic willingness to say yes led to a 2005 contract where Phoenix became the official airline of the CDC. The division was beginning to grow in size but not in scope. The problem was aircraft. Pilots are limited in the number of hours they can fly before stopping for federally mandated crew rest. Phoenix at the time was flying patients in Learjets, which most companies do, but then most companies aren't flying internationally. Because of its small size, there's no room inside a Learjet to carry additional relief crew, which forced them to play a sort of airborne version of leapfrog. Say there's a medevac flight out of Cairo. Phoenix would send one crew on the Learjet to Cairo and a second, by commercial airline, to London. After loading the patient, the Learjet would fly to London where the two crews would swap roles—the first crew would fly home commercially while the second took over patient care inside the Learjet. Sometimes a third crew stationed at yet another airport would also be in play. It was complicated and expensive.

Phoenix had several Gulfstream IIIs by then, which are big enough to carry a second crew. This would've solved the problem, except the Gulfstream III has its own issue. The door. It's too small and poorly situated. You can't get a stretcher through, and even if you did, you wouldn't be able to turn it. The air medical division was stuck in place and suffering from an intractable problem. Or so it seemed until the week before

Christmas of 2004 when Dent and Mark got a call from Bob Tracey. The Danish military had two aircraft they were trying to sell. Gulfstream IIIs. But not just any Gulfstream IIIs. These had a cargo door.

Gulfstream in the 1990s had built six Gulfstream III aircraft with cargo doors for foreign military sales. These were rare and highly specialized aircraft, built quietly and never intended for the domestic market. They didn't even have serial numbers. They'd sold three to the Danes, who used them for search and rescue off the coast of Greenland; two went to the Indian military, which used them to spy on Pakistan; and one was in Saudi Arabia as medevac for the royal family. The brothers were stunned. A business class jet with a cargo door was unheard of. Nobody had one. And with their size, their range, that massive cargo door in the side, they could do anything. This was the break their medical division desperately needed, the *aha* moment when everything would change. But they had to move fast. People were already lining up to grab the airplanes. With the holidays coming up, Phoenix sensed an opportunity.

Most of the interested companies and governments were shutting down for the season and told the Danes they'd negotiate after the new year. Tracey wanted to move now. He asked Dent and Mark to authorize the purchase without ever having seen them. In fact, he was already negotiating with the Danes—all he needed was the money. So they gave it to him. It's the sort of thing a larger company could never do. A week later Mark, Dent, and Bob were in Copenhagen picking up two aircraft so unique and adaptable that, to keep them from falling into the hands of criminals, the Danish military forced them to sign a deal promising not to resell the planes.

The cargo door changed everything. Their air medical operations exploded overnight. And really, anything could be loaded through the door and hauled across the world. They moved enormous fish between aquariums and wolves across continents. Their two Gulfstream IIIs were in such demand that they needed more. They bought a third—the aircraft Dent purchased over the phone, on an island, in his bathing suit, from the Royal Saudi Air Force—and they wanted more. But there were no more. Of the remaining three, one had crashed and two were destroyed in a roof collapse during a heavy snowstorm. Phoenix owned the only three surviving cargo door Gulfstream IIIs on the planet. And Gulfstream wasn't making any more of them. So they decided to make their own.

Which sounds so much easier than it is. The cargo door itself, just the door, has nearly three thousand parts. And then there's the not so minor detail of cutting a massive hole into the side of an aircraft. Once you've done that, you can't just stick a door in there and move on. It's a radical modification. Breaking the structural integrity of an airplane's fuselage decreases its overall strength and that lost strength has to be re-created somehow, redistributed across the rest of the aircraft, to the ceiling, the floor, the opposite side. The airplane cannot fly without such adjustments. They reached out to Gulfstream for specs and an aeronautical engineering company for the design. Then, with the blueprint in hand, they created an in-house aircraft modification department to do the actual work. In perhaps the most Phoenix move of all, placed in charge of this newly formed group and its dizzyingly complicated task was Michael Carter, a civil engineer whose previous job was heading up a municipal water and sewer department.

What do you even call a decision like that—unconventional doesn't begin to cover it. But it's all part of the alchemy of Phoenix Air's success. Believing a skydiving instructor can fly high explosives around the world or that a marketing guy for the cigarette industry can create from whole cloth an international medevac operation that will eventually be run by a middle-aged Mennonite from Indiana—there's an informality and lack of pretense that's born from the philosophy of a company started by two brothers who weren't recognized as experts by the establishment, and it never let that stop them. Because of its origins and outlook, its devil-may-care approach to doing the undoable, Phoenix has always been underestimated. No surprise the people they turn to for solutions have often been underestimated themselves. It's the only way a company from nowhere can find itself, suddenly, everywhere.

Private companies, public institutions, agencies from within the US government, they heard the stories about Phoenix Air—*a suitcase nuke!*—and sent representatives to hear what this little band of pirates in North Georgia could do for them. One of these visitors was Dr. William Walters. As director of Operational Medicine over at the Department of State he was fresh off his dealings with Dent during the Sochi Olympics and now, in the spring of 2014, came to see what in his mind was just another government contractor.

Which was never how Dent saw himself. Visits were never just visits. It was the Disney Scuba Club newsletter all over again. Opportunity waiting to be seized. He led Walters through Phoenix's offices and then across the two-lane road for a tour of the runway and the hangars where aircraft were modified to the exacting, thousandth-of-a-centimeter standards of aviation safety. Hours ticked by as Dent talked with

Walters, rattling off statistics, specs, dates, capabilities, a universe of facts—both those he remembered and the ones he couldn't and just fudged. His arms crossing, uncrossing, eyebrows dancing across his expansive forehead, telling stories in a voice that's serious one minute—he's mortuary-straight when discussing aircraft regulations—and the next erupting into a high-pitched squeal of excitement before plateauing into a satisfied drawl: "You can't make this shit up!"

The last stop on the tour was an unmarked storage room and as he rolled back the massive steel door, Dent motioned for Walters to look inside. Loaded onto the shelves were a half-dozen massive bundles, each about the size of a Cape buffalo. Dent stepped back so Walters could take in the bewildering majesty of this unexpected sight. Walters was a career military man and a doctor, the leader of a group charged with rescuing sick and injured Americans from remote and possibly dangerous areas and then bringing them safely home for treatment. His was a world of questions with no obvious answers, but he had no context for what he was looking at.

Not that it mattered. Because there was Dent—a salesman forever closing—speaking a mile a minute, conjuring federal agencies and life and death stakes, ingenious design, zero gravity test flights, and the repeated failures and ultimate success whose combined result was the equipment stacked and catalogued before them. Each of these bundles represented a capability unavailable anywhere else on planet Earth—the option to transport, by air, patients suffering from the most feared and deadly viruses ever discovered. Airborne, bloodborne, whatever. All without risk to the pilots, crew, or any country whose airspace they entered. Walters was in the presence of a unicorn.

But he didn't need this particular unicorn, not now, which didn't bother Dent in the least. His professional life had given him a unique perspective on time. The journey of Phoenix was less as an arc than a slowly tightening spiral, and each mission established them as the answer to the next question, usually before it was even asked. You never knew when you'd be called upon. He rolled the door shut and clapped on the padlock. Walters left that day without giving the bundles another thought. They were only useful if you were dealing with something deadly and contagious, something that threatened to spread out across the world and endanger the American mainland. And in that moment, in the spring of 2014, no virus like that was on the horizon.

PART TWO

6

Dr. Linda Mobula was poring over lab results in her office when the phone rang. For months now she'd been in Ghana, studying diabetes in the presence of high blood pressure and at last the fieldwork was done. All that remained was to analyze the data; after that she could go back home to the US. Or anyway that was the plan. She didn't know it, but everything was about to change. This was how opportunity and danger, how life itself, tended to arrive for Linda—without warning and sometimes through a side door. Linda was a doctor and researcher and humanitarian who'd lived on two continents and worked on a third; though only thirty-four she'd already earned entrance to prestigious universities and professional networks and global organizations that many people, much older people, only dreamed about. And yet along the way, her education and career, even her childhood, had repeatedly been interrupted, influenced, or radically transformed by pathogens, rebels, and natural disasters. It was an exciting way to live but taxing. She was ready for a break.

It'd been a long year. A long several years. There was medical school at UC San Francisco followed by a residency at Johns Hopkins that was interrupted in the first year by the 2010 earthquake in Haiti. By then Linda had already done fieldwork in the Democratic Republic of Congo and knew global health was her primary interest, and so, putting her residency on hold, she flew to Port-au-Prince and spent months working in a small clinic in the densely populated enclave of Cité Soleil. A bad situation became more so when cholera swept through the area. Linda stayed on, treating families, running the clinic, fighting the outbreak, and eight months later when she returned to Baltimore, it was as a woman experienced beyond her years or education. She finished her residency, got a master's in public health, and completed a fellowship in internal medicine. Not long after that she was in Ghana.

Her work there was almost done and she was set to return home where she already had a new job lined up at USAID that was set to begin in the fall. But first, before that, she planned to take a little time for herself. Just to recover. And now this call. Linda answered in a soft, measured voice, the voice of someone who believes fact is what the data proves it to be. Someone scientific. And yet, bubbling beneath it and bursting from its sides, is the ripple of a laugh that's partially, only half-heartedly, contained. It's somehow a voice that remains steady in the glare of furious action but is also, improbably, exuberant.

The voice on the other end of the line was simply desperate.

The caller was Lance Plyler, a doctor Linda had met the year before in the Philippines. After Typhoon Haiyan, which had wiped out much of the healthcare infrastructure, they'd worked together as part of an international team treating the local population while the country rebuilt itself around them. Lance was now in Liberia, serving as disaster response team leader for Samaritan's Purse, an NGO run by Franklin Graham, which helped to staff and run a hospital in the capital city of Monrovia. The hospital was a finger in the dam in the best of times, but an Ebola outbreak was sweeping the city and Lance's tiny crew of local and foreign doctors was being overrun. They needed help, Lance said, and a doctor of Linda's caliber and experience would be invaluable, if she could come. But no, she couldn't, she needed a break, she needed to go home, or on vacation maybe, to gather herself before starting this new job with USAID and—

"Linda. We need you."

Linda stood there holding the phone. She didn't

want to go but felt compelled to. Not because she'd worked with Ebola or even understood it—in 2014 almost no one had or did—but because of the curses and blessings passed down through generations, those incidental inheritances that become birthright. Linda was born in the US but her parents were from northwest Zaire, the same province where in 1976 the Ebola virus first appeared. She was nine when the family returned, and she was in high school when Ebola erupted in the riverfront town of Kikwit, just 250 miles from their home in Kinshasa. Her adolescence was marked by the wars and coups that transformed Zaire into the Democratic Republic of Congo, a cycle of violence that, for Linda, was punctuated in 1998 when at eighteen she spent several days trapped in her house while rebels attacked the city. Yes, she was a doctor and an American citizen and at times had lived a life of incredible privilege, but she also understood the fear and misery of falling victim to violence and disease. She knew what it was to be helpless—which surely Liberians felt at that moment. She'd been educated at the world's best universities and also hardened by its worst conditions. She was no longer a scared child hiding at home, but among the few people on Earth trained to fight back. Without knowing this outbreak was coming, without ever saying its name, Linda had spent her entire adult life positioning herself to do something about Ebola should it reemerge. And now it was here. She said yes.

It was the rainiest July anyone in Liberia could remember, like the outbreak had arrived on the back of its own weather system. Linda's plane touched down at Roberts International Airport, bounced over the potholes then taxied to the single-story main terminal. She grabbed her bag, stepped into a waiting car, and was swept into the chaos of a capital city under siege. Linda had worked through the aftermath of earthquakes and typhoons, had seen the effects of cholera and malaria and conflict, and she knew Liberia was struggling to overcome a bitter civil war, but Monrovia, home to more than a million people, was worse than anything she'd experienced or expected. Ebola had arrived in the spring. It first appeared in the border areas and villages, far away, but after months of rumors and whispers and the hope (false, as it turned out) that a few weeks without a reported case meant the virus had burnt itself out, Ebola hit the city like a cresting wave. This strain—called Zaire, named for its place of origin—was said to kill 70 percent of its victims. But here in Monrovia, under the right conditions, it killed closer to 90 percent. The month before, one of the city's three hospitals had been completely abandoned after an outbreak. Quietly, quickly, the virus spread. It had found the perfect home.

Liberia was founded on the west coast of Africa in the 1820s by free and formerly enslaved Black Americans. They laid roots and formed a government based on the US constitution, but Africans were already living in Liberia and along the line drawn between these two groups sprang a caste system. People of American descent ruled and everyone else was on the bottom. This disparity planted seeds of bitterness that moldered for 160 years before blossoming into all-out violence in 1989. Liberia's brutal civil war lasted until 2003 and killed hundreds of thousands of people. Even after peace, after the election of President Ellen Johnson Sirleaf, the first female leader of an African nation, prosperity was hard to find. The country had been devastated and much of its professional class had fled. Healthcare was almost nonexistent. In the US there are 2.5 doctors for every one thousand people. That ratio drops in Liberia—a land often called the fever coast—to a terrifying 0.01 doctors per thousand.

By the time the Ebola outbreak struck in 2014, Liberians had already been traumatized by war and its natural resources had been fleeced by multinational corporations. Ebola was just the latest marauder. This history had eroded trust in foreign governments, local government, any government. People didn't trust outsiders or even insiders, didn't trust anyone from beyond their own neighborhood—and in some cases from beyond their own families. Mistrust led to fear and fear to death. Witness Joseph Gbembo—nobody, everybody, a young man from Monrovia. At the start of the outbreak, he attended a public health lecture about handwashing and social distancing, safe handling of the ill and feverish, of the dying, the dead. He carried the knowledge back home, but his family didn't believe him because they didn't believe the experts, especially the foreign experts. Didn't believe Ebola was real. His older brother Prince died first. His corpse was placed in a body bag and carried away by a government team who showed up in white suits and sprayed the whole place down. They came too late. Joseph quickly lost his mother, his aunt, and his nephew. Another brother died, another nephew, his sister, and his brother's wife. Another uncle. Another aunt. In total he lost seventeen members of his family.

When Linda's plane touched down, the worst hadn't even arrived yet, but it was on its way. The capital was terrorized by wailing sirens. Each passing ambulance announced another dead neighbor, one more body to place upon the fires that by now glowed constantly in the night sky. Monrovia had become a haunted place.

ELWA Hospital is located on Monrovia's far western edge and serves as the centerpiece of a 130-acre compound originally constructed in 1951 by the flamboyantly named Christian ministry Eternal Love Winning Africa. Linda pulled through the gates and was struck by the sudden and disorienting sense of calm. No crowded streets, no cars, just grass dotted with palm trees running to a beach slammed flat by ocean waves. She was dropped at the guest house, unpacked, and then set out along the footpath for the five-minute walk to the hospital and its small annex building, the Ebola treatment center, or ETC. ELWA was funded by foreign NGOs such as Samaritan's Purse, the organization that brought Linda to Liberia, but it operated under a spirit of partnership. The hospital's medical director, the forty-six-year-old Jerry Brown, was Liberian, as were many of the physicians and most of the nurses. The hospital had survived years of conflict and upheaval through a sense of local ownership and the city's collective memory of the thousands born and saved there. But goodwill can't defy the elements forever. When Linda arrived, the hospital was decades old and becoming decrepit.

She met Lance Plyler at the hospital and from there he took her to the ETC—a grand name for what in fact was a small chapel recently converted to an isolation unit. Unlike the hospital proper, which Linda found surprisingly calm and well-ordered, the ETC was charged with the unmistakable energy of desperate labor. The footpath leading to the entrance ended in an open-air drying area for used aprons that had been disinfected and were hung from clothes lines. Crooked rows of disinfected rubber boots stood upside down on stakes, and at a glance looked like legs sprung free from shallow graves. Another physician, Nathalie MacDermott, had just finished her rotation in the ETC and stood on the small concrete pad that served as a decon point while staff sprayed her down with a bleach mixture so her boots, gloves, goggles, and full body hooded Tyvek suit could safely be removed. Between the heat and the bleach, ELWA Hospital's determined but clearly improvised response to a ferocious killer, Linda was reeling, almost dizzy. Her introduction only got worse from there.

Along with Nathalie, Lance began to lay out the stark reality of their situation. The converted chapel behind them, capable of holding fewer than a half-dozen patients at a time, had briefly represented the only Ebola treatment unit in southern Liberia. So they'd also converted a storage area into a twenty-bed isolation unit, but that too had filled up immediately. The ELWA staff hadn't signed on for this and weren't set up for it, certainly weren't trained in Ebola response, but they held the line because after them there was no one else. They were providing not a cure but comfort—the survival rate in the first few weeks of the outbreak hovered around 5 percent—and the number of patients was expanding and soon would explode. Doctors and nurses worked their regular shifts in the hospital and then did rotations in the ETC. They were exhausted and scared. That they'd held on even this long was a testament to their collective sense of mission and compassion, a refusal to abandon their patients. But they'd begun to feel abandoned themselves. No governments were stepping in to help, and repeated attempts to alert the international community had gotten no response. The only other organization fighting the outbreak was Doctors Without Borders, known everywhere by their French acronym MSF for Médecins Sans Frontières, but they were so busy elsewhere that they left Monrovia in the hands of the overworked ELWA staff. They were alone and no one else was coming.

And that wasn't all. Lance pulled Linda aside and confided to her that their small staff had just gotten smaller. The doctor in charge of the ETC, an American named Kent Brantly, had come down with a fever and was quarantined at home. They weren't talking about it yet, and no one was sure what he had because bloodwork was pending, but it didn't look good. A volunteer was sick as well, Nancy Writebol, another American, who'd been helping the doctors suit up before their rotations and then running decon once they got out. Her illness was also unknown, Lance said, but maybe, with any luck, it was only malaria.

Because Linda had just arrived, Lance told her to take the night to settle in. She could begin work in the morning. She walked alone to the guest house, past the beach and the storm-tossed sea, wondering what she was doing. She was supposed to be home or on vacation, anywhere but here. She came because she thought she was ready for this but realized now just how wrong she'd been. Malaria, cholera, Haiti, Ghana, Democratic Republic of Congo, the Philippines, nothing had prepared her for this. The situation was spinning out of control and she'd just wandered right in the middle of it. Tomorrow she would crawl inside a plastic suit and step into the crowded chapel to treat a deadly virus she didn't understand at all. A little fear was normal, healthy even, but as Linda reached the guest house and closed the door behind her, what she felt was not healthy fear but terror.

7

Though she didn't yet know it, Linda Mobula had stepped into the rapidly mushrooming epicenter of the deadliest Ebola outbreak in human history. When she arrived in Monrovia in July 2014, the world's understanding of Ebola, even among its experts, was dangerously limited and generally amounted to a sort of pop culture villain that liquifies its victims inside their own skin. Ebola is horrible and horrifying, but it's not a cartoon. Blood doesn't spray or pour or necessarily even weep from your eyes. What you can expect, though, is a rapid and painful death with a terribleness made more terrible still by the fact that it will probably also kill the people you love. Because that's who will be there with you in the end as you lay dying, when Ebola is at its most dangerous.

Ebola has been described as a viral hemorrhagic fever, which is accurate but accounts for only one of the ways it might kill you. What's truly scary is that it can prey on multiple cell types—liver, throat, intestines, whatever—and so death more often comes from a cascading failure of organ systems. The experience reads like a wish list from hell. Abdominal pain, fever, headache, sore throat, nausea and vomiting, loss of appetite, joint pain, muscle pain, chest pain. You'll be too weak to walk, too weak to stand, too weak even to roll away from the mess pouring out of you. Loss of fluid through sweat and puke and diarrhea will quickly bottom out your blood pressure, which has immediate and debilitating effects on the brain. Dying of Ebola often means dying confused or agitated or in a coma-like stupor. If your condition gets serious enough, your eyes will get red but not necessarily hemorrhage—though probably you'll vomit blood. You may have rectal bleeding and bleeding from the gums, and since the virus reduces coagulability, you may also bleed uncontrollably from the very IV punctures meant to replace your disappearing fluids. This loss of clotting factors can be widespread and cause blood to seep from the capillaries and pool beneath the skin, where it's visible as blue and purple bruising. Or maybe the opposite will happen and massive amounts of clots will form—it's a schizophrenic enemy—and block blood flow to the kidneys or the liver, which aside from being incredibly painful will also be in a hurry to kill you. In people who are sick enough, that 90 percent of patients in Monrovia, rapid breathing and hiccups are late and ominous signs.

Ebola is one of the rare viruses able to leap from animals to humans but must be spread deliberately. Blood, sweat, vomit—any infected fluid, really—must enter the body through an opening. The eyes or nose, a cut however small. This makes it seem less transmissible than measles or the flu, but Ebola's parlor trick is its unimaginably high concentration. A milliliter of HIV-infected blood carries one hundred thousand copies of the virus; in Ebola that number reaches into the *billions.* And only a couple of those billions are required for transmission. A drop of sweat in a taxi, a splash of vomit in a vendor's stall, maybe a smear of blood on a door handle—practically just the memory of blood on the door handle—can make you sick. And that tiny amount of fluid that got you sick is all that's required for you to make someone else sick. And on and on and on.

No one knows how long Ebola had been hiding among us, maybe forever, but it began killing in 1976. One day it'd never been detected anywhere and then the next it was inexplicably and almost simultaneously in both Sudan and Zaire. Why and how this happened remains uncertain, but it bears mentioning that humanity had begun intruding on parts of the world previously left alone. Either way, Ebola seemed simply to spring from the earth, a killer without progenitor in modern medical history. Sudan's outbreak—284 infected, 151 killed—came first, but the virus was named for what it did in Zaire. On a rainy night in September 1976, a woman by the name of Sembo Ndobe, hemorrhaging and in labor, appeared at the Yambuku Mission Hospital, a remote Catholic outpost surrounded by forest and dense vegetation. Neither mother nor child survived delivery. More deaths followed. Dozens and then hundreds more, all from the same brutal but mysterious virus. By the time experts arrived at this tiny village on the banks of the Ebola River, the outbreak had burned itself out but only because there was no one left to infect. What little information epidemiologists were able to glean pointed not only to something deadly, but something brand new.

After the twin crises of 1976, Ebola popped up in 1977, then again in 1979. It disappeared in the 1980s—how?, to where?—only to return repeatedly throughout the 1990s and early 2000s. Outbreaks varied in size but often ranged from 200 to 400 cases. Occasionally fatality rates would drop to somewhere near 50 percent but not always. A 2002 outbreak in Democratic Republic of Congo killed 128 of the 143 people infected. As a killer it was murderously efficient, cloaked in mystery and scientific in nature. Think Jack the Ripper sneaking into third period biology. While it had appeared nearly twenty times in less than forty years, by 2014 Ebola remained only partially understood. We knew (kind of) how it spread but not really how to treat it. There was no vaccine, and worse, no cure. There just wasn't enough data, mainly because outbreaks had struck small, isolated populations and quickly ran through the available supply of hosts before going back underground. In short, we'd been getting lucky.

From just this partial view a theory developed: Ebola struck remote places and rendered its victims so sick so fast it was considered unlikely, maybe even impossible, that the infected could make the difficult journey to larger, more populated areas. In other words, Ebola was a self-limiting threat. The problem with this theory was that it ignored the one thing we knew for certain—that once Ebola disappeared there was no way to predict when or where it would strike next.

It began in the Guinean village of Meliandou near the end of 2013. The first patient was a two-year-old boy named Emile. He got it from a fruit bat or a flying mouse or the bite of a bat fly, or maybe from tasting a piece of fruit contaminated by infected saliva or guano. From there it wasn't long until the black diarrhea started—a strong indicator of lower GI bleeding—and within days he was dead. This was late December. By the beginning of 2014 his sister had died and so had his mother and grandmother. Meliandou is a small village, just a couple dozen houses, and even though it's in West Africa, where Ebola had never previously been detected, this outbreak in many ways fit the pattern. But there were important differences. Like how deforestation connected villages with towns and cities and how the people living in them moved quickly along roads and rivers that branched out in all directions. Travel was easy. The funeral for Emile's grandmother alone attracted mourners from miles around. They left home, entered a village where Ebola was active, sat with her body (still contagious), and then returned to their families and friends as unknowing accomplices to a killer.

One of those accomplices was the midwife who'd taken care of her, who got sick, who traveled to Gueckedou—a city of two hundred thousand—and died in a local hospital. One of *her* caretakers got infected and she too traveled, going nearly sixty miles for treatment in Macenta. That's how fast it happened. Transmission requires only contact and time, and Ebola was now in multiple villages, multiple cities, loose among hundreds of thousands of people, each of them talking, touching, sharing the same space, traveling even—by bike, by taxi, across rivers and borders—carrying the virus farther with each step. Cases popped up sporadically and at great distances from each other, so doctors failed to recognize them as early markers of the same rapidly spreading outbreak. They didn't even recognize the culprit. This wasn't Sudan or DRC or Uganda, it was Guinea—Ebola couldn't exist here. It was mistaken for malaria or Lassa fever, anything but what it really was.

It moved and it stalked, it grew, and it happened so quietly that no one noticed. It wasn't until February that reports surfaced of a strange illness wiping out entire communities. Another month passed while an international team of doctors and epidemiologists from Guinea, Sierra Leone, France, Germany, and Belgium studied samples of infected blood. It was mid-March when they alerted the World Health Organization headquarters in Geneva that the mystery pathogen—a mystery no more—was Ebola.

The CDC dispatched a team of investigators who concluded that the virus was contained. This was the majority opinion, based on what had happened in the past and what appeared now to be happening on the ground. But this opinion didn't properly account for two key factors—geography and demographics.

Guinea, Sierra Leone, and Liberia share long and porous borders and have large, urban populations. Guinea's capital city alone is home to 1.6 million people. And they're mobile. All three countries have large international airports serving worldwide destinations. As MSF would later note, Ebola had found not just a new home, but maybe the perfect home.

8

Hundreds of miles and another country away, Dr. Kent Brantly was at his house on the ELWA compound when an email popped up on his computer. Picture Kent: Twenty-seven. Wiry. The sort of piercing blue eyes and perfectly trimmed beard that demand to be described—no doubt to the horror of someone dedicated to service and austerity—as Hollywood. He was also a family medicine physician who, along with his wife, Amber, had felt called by God to serve in foreign missions. He'd already practiced medicine in South America and East Africa, and most recently had worked at Mulago Hospital in Uganda. It'd only been a few months since he and Amber and their two young children arrived at ELWA, but already Kent was making a mark. He was determined, smart, skilled, and seemed to have endless compassion for his patients. Along with his regular duties, he'd been placed in charge of ELWA's HIV task force. The email he received that afternoon was from another of the ELWA doctors, a surgeon from Oregon, passing along news that Ebola had been confirmed in Guinea and was suspected in Sierra Leone:

"It's a bit close for comfort. We all need to be alert to the possibility of seeing something here."

This was March 22, 2014. Two days later the medical staff met for a discussion on how to prepare and execute a plan should Ebola become something more than a possibility. This felt to Kent like an overreaction—two days ago the virus wasn't on his radar and even now felt like a distant and toothless assailant. But the more he listened to the horrors unfolding in Guinea the more precarious their own situation appeared—whatever conditions had combined to create an explosive outbreak there also existed here. The journey from "totally unaware" to "completely prepared" would be a steep climb dogged by unanswered questions. Of these the biggest question was where. ELWA's main hospital had no place to quarantine highly infectious patients. They'd have to find someplace else to put the Ebola treatment center. Ultimately, someplace else ended up being that small chapel on the ELWA grounds that would yield nothing larger than a five-bed facility.

There were also the risks to manage. Given Liberia's already low ratio of citizens to doctors—the ratio was better in both Guinea and Sierra Leone but just barely—Kent understood that fighting an Ebola outbreak would require many things, not the least of which being the fighters themselves. Protecting the few professionals available to treat patients was of critical importance. Keeping doctors and nurses safe from the virus they were treating would require everyone adhering to a clearly defined and strictly enforced set of protocols. These rules would outline everything from personal protective gear to treatment regimens, on down to how best to sterilize or destroy equipment once it had been used. In a sign of just how uncharted these waters were, not only did ELWA lack Ebola protocols, but the most current guidelines Kent could find were published by the WHO nearly twenty years prior.

This first Ebola meeting at ELWA sparked a frenzy of planning and thinking, but after that there was nothing to do but wait. Normal life continued, but not really. The threat loomed over everything. Kent obsessively checked Twitter for updates from the WHO and the CDC. He watched the outbreak spread and get bigger, get closer. Like the rumble of an invading army that hadn't yet crested the horizon, it wasn't here but they could feel it coming. Then, finally, it hit. A pair of sisters, both infected, arrived at the northwestern border where Liberia collides with Guinea and Sierra Leone. One sister died shortly after crossing. The second made it all the way to Monrovia before succumbing to the virus in a hospital near the airport. As best anyone could tell, she'd had eighty close contacts. Ebola had arrived.

Up to this point, the spread had been relatively slow and often went unnoticed. Now it broke out into the open. By the beginning of April there were hundreds of deaths in Guinea alone. Hotspots spread out across three countries and yet the only people actively combating it were local public health agencies and a handful of NGOs. Calls for help went out but failed to stir action. If and when Ebola came to ELWA, there would be no help. Over the next two weeks, the staff trained and prepared their response—proper use of personal protective equipment, how to handle dead bodies, how to mix the bleach solution that would disinfect everything from dirty equipment to the ground patients walked upon. The chapel was formally converted into an ETC, fences were built. Latrines were dug and water pipes laid.

Pressure mounted. In May, a group of foreign volunteers working in Guinea were attacked by villagers who believed they were the ones spreading Ebola. That same month violence came to ELWA when a man with symptoms of an unknown hemorrhagic fever—it turned out not to be Ebola—died in the ER. A crowd gathered and demanded the body, which ELWA's staff had placed in a coffin. Kent feared the public handling and burial of an infected body would only further spread the disease and he asked why they would even consider handing the body over.

"Because they're threatening to kill us," another doctor said. "They're threatening to burn down the hospital and kill all of us, and it's not worth it."

A crisis was averted when the cops came and took the body directly to the family's burial site. But the reprieve was temporary. Fear and confusion are willing accomplices to violence. When the flu pandemic of 1918 hit Philadelphia, local leadership so thoroughly botched the response that the city erupted in chaos and violence. The same was happening now. In the absence of knowledge, the imagination takes over. And the mind produces only monsters.

Everything was happening very fast. By June, West Africa's first outbreak was already the worst in history, and more people were getting sick all the time. The few remaining hospitals not yet overrun or abandoned announced they weren't equipped to treat Ebola patients and refused to admit them. This left ELWA as the only hope in a desperate city. On Wednesday, June 11, with anxiety running high, their first patient arrived. She showed up with her uncle in an ambulance. The uncle was dead before he made it inside. The young woman lived a few days and appeared to improve, then took a sudden turn, became unresponsive, and died. The staff was left gasping. Between the long process of getting into and out of PPE, the constant disinfecting, the helplessness of watching a patient slowly die before their very eyes, not to mention the all-consuming worry of getting infected themselves—when it was all tallied up, just one Ebola patient had pushed them to the edge of their capabilities. The coming wave, if and when it came, would sweep them away.

When it came to Ebola the reality on the ground defied definition. And anyway, the definitions themselves were always changing. Rumor and conjecture passed for fact. The virus was a new kind of Ebola or not even Ebola. It was malaria or Lassa fever. It was fake; it was gone; it was spread by food, by magic. Meanwhile, people kept dying in what had been called an outbreak but sounded increasingly, to the few experts listening, like an epidemic. ELWA's five-bed treatment center became swamped and dangerous, so a storage area was converted to a twenty-bed facility. It opened on July 20. Kent was placed in charge, and that day he received thirteen patients. The following day eight more came. With more patients came more dying.

There was the woman who tried to reach ELWA by taxi but died before arrival. A mother and daughter walked in together then died separately. Family members showed up and sat outside, waiting for news only to become sick themselves.

Patients died slowly, painfully. Sweating and vomiting, with constant diarrhea. Feverish and in pain, entirely aware of what was happening one minute, confused and agitated the next. It was death by suffering, by constant evacuation. Each death was marked by how miserable and graphic it was. And just about all of them died. Corpses were sprayed with bleach, wrapped in plastic, and then carried off by the Ministry of Health to mass graves. Eventually this too became inefficient and that's when the cremations started. ELWA's lone survivor during this time was a fourteen-year-old named Gebah, the miracle patient who lay for days as eyewitness to hell.

To lose nearly every patient who walked, crawled, or was carried through the door demoralized everyone. Kent fought against the creeping defeatism by reminding himself that they weren't just treating people but comforting them as well, lessening the loneliness and humiliation that is death by Ebola. He'd kicked a soccer ball with Gebah, and with the others he held hands, aware that clad in his PPE all they could see were his eyes. Aware, too, that his were the eyes of a stranger, a foreigner, which only added to their sense of isolation, regardless of his intentions. But still he tried. He worked shifts in the hospital, his regular shifts, the shifts he'd come here to work, and then made his way to the ETC. As the patient count rose so did the need for staff, and into this breach stepped Nancy Writebol, fifty-nine, another American, who volunteered to work the dressing and decon stations. Nancy's job was to mix the bleach solution used to clean boots and goggles and aprons, which was sprayed on door handles and railings and walkways, anything that was touched in any way by the infected or those who treated them.

When Kent arrived outside the ETC for a shift, it was Nancy who greeted him. She would help get him into his PPE, and as she taped his gloves over the sleeves of his gown, she'd call out—as a reminder of the stakes and her own need to be careful—the names of Kent's children. *This one's for Stephen, this one's for Ruby.* When he came out, she'd be there waiting. Spraying him with bleach and calling out the steps for the safe removal of PPE, which was as dangerous as anything else because it's here, when you're exhausted, that a mistake is made. Everything they were doing took concentration, but everyone was so tired and so stressed that a mistake would've seemed inevitable if there'd been time to stop and think about it. Which there wasn't.

Kent was doing what everyone was doing at ELWA, and on a good day he was working sixteen to eighteen hours. Sometimes he'd go to work at seven in the morning and not return until noon the next day, sleep an hour, wake up to phone calls from the hospital, and go back in. He wasn't eating nearly enough for the hours he put in and between that and the stress, not to mention the heat, he lost thirty pounds. Amber was worried, and Kent too wanted to stop, but stopping meant leaving that much more work to the already overworked staff. It was around this time that Amber and the kids went back to the US for a wedding. It was just as well, because a couple days after they left, on July 23, Kent woke with a temperature of 100. It was elevated but below the 100.4 threshold for screening patients for Ebola, and so he told himself it was something he'd eaten or malaria or the exhaustion. Still, he called out sick. That afternoon Lance Plyler came over. Just to be safe, just to rule it out, just because they were living and practically drowning in it, Lance tested Kent for Ebola. They didn't yet know it, but Nancy was also sick. Thirty miles away, Linda Mobula's plane touched down at Roberts International Airport.

9

There's a moment that first morning in a foreign place when you wake up to a world so new and disorienting that for a minute you don't know where you are. Then, slowly, the mind catches up and you remember. Excitement splashes in, there's wonder and adventure. Unless the place you're waking up to is Liberia of 2014. Unless you're in the ELWA guest house and the reason you're there is to join an outmatched crew of doctors overrun by a spiraling Ebola epidemic. Because then what you're waking up to is fear. That first day, and every day after, Linda Mobula woke up to fear.

There was the fear of what she knew but also what she didn't. Ebola was a wasteland of the unknown. In 2011, when she was fighting cholera in Haiti, convoys of trucks would arrive at the clinic to drop off a hundred-odd patients at a time. It was overwhelming but it wasn't frightening because doctors have been treating cholera for two hundred years. Ebola had no such history. There was only a scattered understanding of what to do, and that was overshadowed by questions of why it was spreading so fast. Ebola wasn't thought to be airborne but a number of people, smart people who for decades had been working with infectious disease, were talking about how this strain was much more virulent than anything they'd seen in the past. They assumed it had mutated. And if the virus itself had changed, then maybe how it spread changed also. Maybe it was airborne. Linda didn't think so but she also didn't know. To find out you'd need to study a representative sample size—what scientists call the N. But too little research had been done to conduct a meaningful study. The N wasn't big enough. She didn't know for certain, and that uncertainty scared her. Scared her enough to think *What am I doing here?*, scared her enough to think *I'm not ready for this*. Scared her so much that in a photo taken during those first hours you can actually see in her eyes just how scared she really was.

That morning, she left the guest house and made the five-minute walk to the new twenty-bed ETC in the storage area. A security guard sat out front and behind him was a handwritten sign: *Stay Away! Isolation unit. Authorized personnel only.* She entered the dressing area in scrubs and was helped into full PPE—Tyvek suit, rubber boots, and two pairs of gloves, the outer pair taped over the sleeves of the suit. Then came the plastic apron, surgical mask, goggles, and a modified hood that went from the top of her head all the way down to her shoulders, front and back. There was a lot of pulling on and cinching down and tying up. This process alone could take thirty minutes. Fully dressed and sealed, the temperature inside the suit rose to 115 degrees. She had trouble hearing or seeing or even moving. Sitting on someone's bed, holding their hand, providing personal care—these things were all but impossible. Doctors going in wrote their names with a Sharpie on the front of their Tyvek suits to lessen the anonymity, but the patients were living and dying in extreme isolation.

The United States Army Medical Research Institute of Infectious Diseases, USAMRIID, located on the Ft. Detrick Army base in Frederick, Maryland, is where the US government houses and studies dangerous pathogens. Ebola is kept in a small suite of negative pressure rooms known by the designation AA-05. Entering suite AA-05 is not easy. You begin in a locker room where you strip off your clothes and put on a clean pair of scrubs. From the locker room you enter into Level 2. When that door opens the first thing you notice is the slight draw of air against your clothes from the negative pressure meant to keep anything on the inside from escaping to the outside. On entering you move through a blue ultraviolet light that breaks down any viruses on your body, hampering their ability to replicate. Inside you put on a pair of clean, white socks and enter Level 3. Inside is a desk and makeshift chair where the next set of protective gear is donned. There's a bottle of baby powder, which you shake onto your hands before slipping on surgical gloves, and a roll of tape to secure both the cuffs of the gloves to the ends of your sleeves and the top of your socks to the bottom of your pant legs. Next you climb into a full-body rubberized biohazard suit and pull the hood over your head. Once the hood is zipped tight, you connect an air hose to fill the suit and then move through yet another airlock to Level 4. Your boots are here and once they're on you can move down the corridor, past a series of doors—each leading to a different pathogen—until you reach suite AA-05.

Entering the ELWA Ebola treatment unit was a slightly different experience for Linda. She stood outside in the mud and slipped into a set of PPE so recently used it was still warm. Then she stepped into the treatment area. Her eyes stung from the sweat and her goggles fogged up immediately. Her limited vision went almost to no vision and it was like this—cut off from her senses and weighed down by knee-high rubber boots—that she treated patients. Accepted practice in 2014 was to give antibiotics and antimalarial drugs, electrolytes such as potassium, and fluids. Lots of fluids. If someone is losing large amounts of fluid, mostly you're in a race to replace them. By mouth if possible, but if they're too weak to drink or too sick to keep it down, then you stick them with a needle and give the fluids by IV. So that's what Linda did. Half-blind and through two pairs of gloves, she started IVs on patients suffering from a terrifying disease. Hoping that none of the blood would find its way through a tiny opening in her suit. That she wouldn't stick herself with a dirty needle. Really, it was treatment by approximation: *These are the things we believe might help*. But they might not. She went from bed to bed, checking old IV lines, starting new ones, running fluids, giving meds. In nearly any other hospital, fluids and drugs would be regulated by IV pumps, but ELWA had no IV pumps—nor did they have a lab to run blood work. Drip rates had to be calculated by hand, blood chemistry guessed at by symptom, therapies improvised by outcome.

Shifts inside the ETC were supposed to last less than forty-five minutes but doctors regularly stayed in as long as an hour. Once Linda's shift was over, she began the long process of spraying out. She exited the ETC backward so the bottom of her boots could be sprayed before touching uncontaminated ground. Then her whole body was sprayed down and the dirty PPE was removed one layer at a time. This process ate into precious downtime and when it was finally over and she'd caught her breath, had at last stopped sweating, it was time to go back in. Because there were always more patients. They were coming in faster now, from all over Monrovia with fear in their eyes. Adults, children, nearly all of them facing bad outcomes. That first day she treated a family of six that one by one all died.

It wasn't long before the nightmares started. Mostly that she had Ebola and was feverish. They were so realistic Linda would wake in the middle of the night convinced she was dying and call out to no one: "Oh my God, I have a fever!" She kept a thermometer by the bed and though her temperature never spiked, she was living the nightmare. Even in the light of day there was a creeping hysteria brought on by movies like *Outbreak* and *Contagion* and that book *The Hot Zone*. All this had left an impression that the medical staff couldn't shake. In this pop culture version of the virus—Ebola's evil twin—where blood shoots from your eyes and your body is liquified, the pathogen mutates and turns global, turns the whole world into a postapocalyptic waste zone, and in that worst-case reality their tiny island in this angry sea would be ground zero.

And maybe it already was. Kent was sick and

though his first Ebola test came back negative, protocol dictated he needed another clean test before he could be cleared, and the results of that second definitive test weren't in yet. Nor was there official word on Nancy. Some staff had quit and others had finished their rotation and gone home, so even as their patient load was increasing, fewer providers were there to handle it. There'd always been a risk to treating Ebola patients, they all knew that, but they'd always assumed that someone, at some point, would come to their aid. They couldn't stop, nor could they hold on forever. So where was everybody? Linda tried to stay calm, but it was clear that by any objective measure it was almost time to panic.

10

The dam finally broke on Saturday, July 26. Liberian Independence Day. Kent awoke at 2 p.m. to find Dr. John Fankhauser looming over him in full PPE. Lance Plyler stood outside his open bedroom window in street clothes. Kent's lab work had come in. Lance looked him in the eye:

"Kent, bud. We got your test result. I'm sorry to tell you, man. Your test is positive."

Kent stared back. "I really wish you hadn't said that."

That afternoon Lance pulled Linda aside and told her the news. He said that since Kent was alone at home, they'd just isolate him where he was. Linda hadn't yet met Kent, and Lance asked her to take over his care. *But keep it to yourself*, he told her, *the rest of the staff doesn't know yet*. Everyone else found out that night. The idea was to break it gently at the daily staff meeting but as the leadership team stared at their shoes trying to work up the courage to deliver news of a worst-case scenario, Lance's phone chirped with a message. Nancy's test was in. She too had Ebola. It was like someone sucked the air out of the room, like time stopped, like the universe—after ignoring the staff of ELWA all these months—decided to sucker punch them. The overall feeling was nausea. Everyone knew the most likely outcome for Kent and Nancy, but what they didn't know was how it'd come to this in the first place. Kent was the guy in charge, the doctor who designed the protocol—a protocol they'd practiced over and over. No one had been more meticulous than Kent and yet he still got infected. How? When? From which patient? There were no answers, so each question begot another. Had he done something wrong, were they *all* doing something wrong, did PPE even *work*?

Kent was lucky in at least one regard—his family was safely back home in the States. Things were different for Nancy Writebol. Her husband David was still here. David was pulled out of the meeting so he could be informed before everyone else, and then, alone, he walked back to their house. When he got there, he said, "Nancy, we have some really hard things to talk about."

He told her about Kent and that her test had also come back. There's no gentle way to say *you have Ebola* but David did his best. He tried to touch her, to comfort her, but Nancy knew better and held out her hands: "Don't."

Linda stood outside Kent's house and put on her PPE. The staff had made the collective decision that if one of them or even a bunch of them got sick that everyone else would stay, regardless of the risk, that they'd take care of one another. It's one thing to make such a gesture of solidarity in theory but they now faced the reality. As she got ready, Linda thought of Kent's wife and his kids and the very real possibility that he would never see them again. She didn't have a family of her own yet, but it was impossible not to put herself in Kent's shoes and imagine his fate as her own. They were close in age and had similar training. Like her, he had volunteered to serve under impossible conditions and now the worst thing that *could* happen *was* happening. As she stepped over the threshold and went inside, she was thinking that if Kent could get sick then anyone could get sick, and that realization led to maybe the scariest question of all, the one they were all thinking but nobody was asking out loud: *Am I going to die here?*

11

Deep inside a lodge on the remote southern edge of Alaska, Franklin Graham paced his office. Since getting the news he'd racked his brain, he prayed, he lay sprawled across the floor. He didn't know what to do. Beyond the window a pontoon plane bobbed at its mooring. Wind swept across Lake Clark. Samaritan's Purse owns land up in Port Alsworth and runs a retreat for wounded veterans and their spouses. Graham had come to get lost with them in this wilderness but even here the world found him. At first there was just shock but then came fear and confusion, a creeping anxiety that broke the surface in a dizzy swirl of panic. *One of our doctors has Ebola.* Graham founded Samaritan's Purse in 1970, and in the decades since, the organization had grown. He now had missions all over the world. It was dangerous work, the doctors and support staff knew the risks, *he* knew the risks, but from the very start he'd been uneasy about Ebola. He didn't like that members of his staff were treating it, but that spring when MSF asked them to join the fight everyone said yes. Because this was the work they did.

Still. There'd been a knot in his stomach the whole time and now his fears were realized. He stopped pacing, snatched the receiver from his office phone, and called a house three thousand miles away in Abilene, Texas.

Amber Brantly was in her childhood bedroom, crying. Kent had called her after he found out and said simply, "It's positive." They didn't talk for long, maybe both of them were in shock, but as soon as she hung up her parents rushed in. Kent was sick halfway across the world and there was no way she could get to him and even less chance he could get to her. He might *never* get back, might die far from home and by himself. She sat on the bed with her parents as her kids played in the next room. How long they sat there she didn't know but then her phone was ringing, and she answered and a voice over the line was saying, "Amber, this is Franklin Graham."

Graham didn't know what to say. He knew that Ebola was a death sentence. That getting Kent back was just short of impossible. But also Graham knew he had an obligation to try.

"I want you to know that we're going to do everything we possibly can to get your husband back."

It was a promise and he meant it, but he had no idea how to get it done.

Graham left Alaska that day. He flew to his organization's headquarters in Boone, North Carolina where a command post had already been set up and furious around-the-clock work was underway. One of their own was overseas and dying and it weighed heavily on everyone. That and the arc of the virus. If you plot out a timeline of how Ebola kills its victims, the distance from first symptoms to grisly death is only eight days. Kent had already been sick two days. Barring outside intervention or evacuation, some miracle, there was a 90 percent chance Kent Brantly would be dead by Thursday.

There was also Nancy Writebol. She didn't technically work for Samaritan's Purse, wasn't technically Graham's responsibility, but she'd been so much a part of the effort, the misery, the responsibility, helping doctors to gear up and spray out, that the organization decided whatever it took to get Kent, they'd double it and get Nancy too. Outbound phone lines whistled with activity. Their first calls were to insurance companies that carried the organization's emergency evacuation policies, but none of them wanted any part of Ebola and refused to get involved. Graham pushed back. He'd been paying premiums all these years and now he wanted something for it. Their response—*sue us*—left no room for negotiation. He went to the air carriers. Commercial. Private. Anyone he could think of. No's came back so fast you could almost see a roomful of executives staring in horror at a speaker phone, shaking their heads, wondering who had answered this call in the first place, someone finally mumbling *whatcan'thearyoutoomuchstatic* as his assistant pressed the END CALL button. The lone exception was a South African charter company with a 737 who said, "Yeah we can do that, but only for a million dollars a head," and at that point Graham was so desperate he would've considered it if not for this other problem that had just now crept up.

No country would take Kent. This information came through as mosaic but slowly coalesced into immutable fact. Hospitals and consulates and public health officials in cities across North Africa, one after another, said no. Europe, briefly, was a glimmer of hope. MSF had relationships with medical facilities in Brussels and Geneva, so the thinking was maybe Europe might be an option. But the South African charter company didn't have the technology or the staff or the know-how to safely transport Ebola patients, not even for a million dollars. The Europeans weren't particularly enthusiastic about the idea of a plane touching down and the door popping open to reveal not just a hemorrhaging patient, but also a pilot and copilot, a navigator, flight attendants—whoever—all bleeding and about to explode. And it wasn't that they didn't want a plane like that on their runway, they didn't even want a plane like that in their *airspace*. What if something went wrong, a mechanical issue, or an on-board fire, a severe and unexpected storm, some act of God or sabotage that forced the plane to land? The answer was no. Not just from the countries they hoped to fly into but also from those they only wanted to fly over.

This was resistance foretold. Just a few days before, Sheik Umar Khan, a thirty-nine-year-old doctor from Sierra Leone with a shaved head and million-dollar smile, became ill with Ebola after months of leading his country's response to the outbreak. Khan was the steady hand on the ground as the virus exploded across West Africa, the expert that the world's experts turned to for information. He was, for a time, the entirety of the local response and also the nexus of the international response. He was a hero in his homeland, indispensable to the effort, and when news of his diagnosis went public, a massive effort to get him someplace with advanced care quickly spun up. The WHO wanted to fly him to their headquarters in Geneva, but the company they chartered to run the flight took one look at him—the fever, the blood, the vomiting—and said, "No he's too sick, too contagious, won't make it, we'll see ya." Khan remained in Sierra Leone.

So what to do with Kent and Nancy? With Europe and Africa both off the table, there was one option—fly due west over the Atlantic and head straight for the US. It would not be a quiet mission. Once Kent's diagnosis was confirmed, Samaritan's Purse put out a press release that immediately went viral. "The American Doctor with Ebola" was all over the news. A world that until this moment had ignored the outbreak suddenly tuned in and cranked up the volume. There'd be no sneaking him in; they'd have to enter through the front door, which meant the mission would need the full and public support of the American government. Focus shifted to DC. Franklin's father, Billy Graham, was the famous minister who'd counseled every US president from Lyndon Johnson to Barack Obama. The organization had powerful connections in Washington and beyond. Graham turned to Ken Isaacs, his VP of government relations, to find someone who could breathe life into a proposition that everywhere else was dead on arrival.

Isaacs called Sylvia Burwell, secretary of the US Department of Health and Human Services, and Tom Friedan, director of the CDC, to figure out what the protocol was for bringing someone with Ebola into the US. While he waited on an answer, Samaritan's Purse called in every favor they had. They reached out to senators and representatives, to the *aides* for senators and representatives, to department heads, functionaries, people who made decisions, and people who just answered the phone. Everyone was sympathetic and alarmed; it was clear that after months of beating the drum the US government was beginning to awaken to the reality that Ebola could (and probably would) reach our shores. But no one could help. It didn't seem to Graham they particularly wanted to help. Nobody was willing to stick their neck out and risk being the person who infected the American public with Ebola.

And anyway, nobody had the first clue where to start. There was no medical, legal, or logistical precedent for what they were proposing. The CDC wasn't certain the human body under these conditions could even survive the flight. The public health system was overmatched by just two cases of Ebola—twenty-four hours of furious effort hadn't yielded a single person with an idea of how to help them. Hope wasn't entirely gone but the lights were beginning to dim.

12

Dr. William Walters at State was working on two hours of sleep when the call came in. He'd spent the previous day coordinating the evacuation of the US embassy in Tripoli after fighting between rival militias threatened the Americans stationed there. Libya's descent into chaos had been precipitous since 2011 when the government was overthrown as part of the Arab Spring. That had led almost directly to the disaster at Benghazi, and the US government was eager to avoid another Benghazi. With shells landing near and occasionally within the compound walls, the embassy had to be closed and its 158-person diplomatic staff spirited overland across four hundred miles of North African desert in a forty-vehicle convoy protected by five fighter jets and eighty US marines. When they were finally over the border and safely into Tunisia, Walters crawled into bed.

He was barely asleep when the next crisis arose,

delivered over the phone by a nameless staffer for one of the 435 members of the House of Representatives.

"There are two Americans infected with Ebola in West Africa."

Walters sat up in bed. "Okay, you have my attention."

There was a pause over the line. If Walters was waiting for something else—a plan, resources, anything at all—he would've been disappointed because here the conversation shifted and the barrel of responsibility pointed directly back at him.

"I hear you're the person at the State Department who deals with this kind of stuff," the staffer said. "So, what are you going to do about it?"

And there it was. This wasn't a courtesy call or a bringing-you-up-to-speed call. It was a handoff; nobody else was coming. Walters hung up the phone wondering how this had become his life.

That Walters was in his current position could be viewed in one light as accidental and in another as the only outcome possible. William Walters grew up in the Finger Lakes region of western New York and joined the Army out of high school. The military made him a paramedic, then a flight medic. Somewhere along the way they recognized his aptitude for medicine and put him through nursing school, then medical school. He stayed in the Army, took an officer's commission, and served three tours in Iraq as a flight surgeon. He returned to the civilian world, got into air ambulance work, lived a normal life.

Then in 2011 the State Department created a new division, something radically different from anything they'd ever done before. Rather than sending family practice or occupational medicine doctors to embassies, they now wanted physicians who specialized in emergency medicine, people capable of handling everything, including some of the weirder stuff. No one was sure what that weirder stuff would be exactly, just that they might need it. Call it a premonition. Walters was hired as the first director of Operational Medicine in December of 2011, and the attacks on the Americans stationed in Benghazi happened the following September. How that mess shook out for Walters was it lit a fire under State to become much more proactive in the planning and execution of rescue missions, and he was in charge of the group deputized to pull them off.

It didn't take Walters long to recognize State as the perfect place to work if you're the kind of person who likes being handed strange problems. And he is exactly that kind of person. By July 2014 Walters and his team were handling a whole assortment of international dustups, plus the odd extraction of Americans—both government and otherwise—who'd run into trouble overseas. This latest problem was exactly the sort of thing he did.

Walters threw back the sheets and headed downstairs. The pattern of response by now was familiar—phone calls, game plans, coffee. The fog slowly began to lift. He'd only been given the broad strokes of the situation unfolding in Monrovia but they painted a grim picture. Which more or less was Operational Medicine's specialty. But with this particular mission he anticipated pushback. When it came to highly infectious diseases the prevailing wisdom was clear—*You don't bring the zombie apocalypse to a place that doesn't have zombies*. This was gospel to everyone but Walters. He was a veteran and a doctor and had a firm grasp on both the risk and the medicine. And his group had a long track record of marshaling US resources to pull off the impossible—so why not this? There was also the matter of Walters's boss, Under Secretary for Management Pat Kennedy, a career diplomat who knew how to navigate the tricky bureaucratic channels of the federal government. Kennedy had established an environment where, so long as it was legal, moral, and ethical, the people under him could do what they believed they *should* do. It was a rare degree of autonomy within a large bureaucracy that freed Walters to act without asking. Pretty much that's what he was doing now.

Standing in his suburban Virginia house, Walters went through his mental Rolodex of worst-case scenario specialists. This didn't take long—it's a pretty short list of people who don't hang up when you start talking about Ebola. Essentially there was only one name. Walters grabbed his phone.

13

As he sat on his deck that warm afternoon in July 2014, Dent Thompson didn't know if Walters would call him back. Part of him hoped it was over. He'd come up to Beech Mountain to get away from the madness of Phoenix Air, from the constant grind that comes with being the COO and senior vice president of a company whose employees are strung out across the globe doing work for insurance companies and drilling companies, for private individuals, for the government, the military. He was here to kick back and had no plans except to drink this beer. Part of him actually believed that he'd scared Walters off by insisting the government send experts to inspect his equipment in Cartersville. This showed a fundamental misunderstanding of William Walters.

He's simply a different breed. Be it his background, his training, a peculiarity in his disposition or DNA, there's something about Walters that makes him stand out from nearly everyone around him. Yes, the State

Department was a place where you could find yourself involved in strange and dangerous missions but this particular mission was strange and dangerous in all the wrong ways, ways that people had definitely not joined State to handle. Just being involved in it could keep you from getting promoted, and a screw up, however small, well, that would get you fired. But neither of those things bothered Walters in the least. He's wired for results, not rank.

And so, just as Dent started to slip back into the lazy flow of vacation, his phone rang. The 202 area code. Walters again. The United States government had made a decision. Dent, who's never quiet, was quiet when he answered.

"Tuesday morning," Walters said. "We'll have the whole world at your doorstep."

PART THREE

14

Dent and Pepper first met in a bar called Frankie's in the Prado. He made a pass and she laughed at him. Not with him, at him. Important distinction. Dent, being Dent, wasn't bothered at all. He kept on until he won her over, until they became the most perfect of odd couples. But something of that original dynamic remains. Phoenix Air is life for Dent, but Pepper's plans don't involve planes bound for far-off chaos—she is forever changing, evading, or ignoring that subject. She's almost intentionally unimpressed by the stories, like some part of her is still at Frankie's laughing at the self-importance of this man and his business, still waiting for that drink. After the call with Walters, when Dent walked inside to find Pepper and said without ceremony *vacation's over*, you can almost imagine her look of disbelief, the arrival of clouds. The silence (or not) as she packed to go home.

Dent's a worrier by nature and what he faced now was a mission practically looking for ways to fail—failure to secure permits, failure of equipment, failure to keep the patient alive, failure to not contaminate the entire Western Hemisphere with Ebola. This fear of failure wasn't new, it was just heightened and he dealt with it the way he dealt with all his anxieties—by identifying the scariest problem and fixing that first. Inner peace through external action. Right now, atop the list of things eating away at him was the risk Ebola posed to his people. As soon as Dent and Pepper got in the car, he called Dr. Mike.

By 2014 Dr. Mike wasn't just the top doctor for Phoenix's air-medical team, he was the top doctor for all of Phoenix Air. Engineers, mechanics, pilots, secretaries, they came to him with ailments large and small, with routine medical questions, things they didn't discuss even with their wives or husbands. And Dr. Mike would treat them like his own patients because really that's what they were. They looked to him for help and he took that responsibility seriously. Joining him on the call that day was Vance Ferebee, a sixty-one-year-old nurse with a syrupy North Carolina accent. Back in the 1970s Vance dropped out of college, wasn't sure what to do with his life, and just sort of stumbled into nursing. It was still very much a female profession then and he was surrounded by women, which was fine with him. He became a flight nurse and an ICU nurse and joined Phoenix Air in 2003 when the medical division was first formed. Four years later Vance was named the team's manager.

Dr. Mike and Vance would ultimately bear responsibility for deciding, respectively, if and how Phoenix pulled off this mission and Dent was eager to gauge their reactions. The two of them listened as Dent explained what little Walters had told him and also how the whole thing hinged on the upcoming dog and pony show that either would or would not establish them as the only people anywhere with the ability to safely transport Ebola patients. Their participation was entirely voluntary but if the experts liked what they saw at Phoenix Air on Tuesday, pressure to say yes would be immense. Now was the time to express any reservations.

Dr. Mike and Vance were used to flying dangerous missions all over the world. To Gitmo, Somalia, Niger, and the Central African Republic. They flew into dusty airstrips across South America to extract shadowy figures injured in circumstances never convincingly explained. They brought home Otto Warmbier—the American student imprisoned in North Korea for tearing a propaganda poster off a hotel wall—and recently they'd flown into South Sudan during a coup. That one was spicy—soldiers and rebels everywhere, officials in the Pentagon scanning satellite images to make sure none of the combatants got too close to the airport while the Phoenix crew sat exposed and waiting on the tarmac for the arrival of eleven critically injured patients. So they were experienced. But still. This was Ebola. And they'd be the ones trapped with it, for hours, inside the narrow fuselage of a modified Gulfstream III jet. Dent wanted to know, could they do this.

Dr. Mike spoke for both of them. "Sure," he said, with the casual shrug, a gesture that started with Mark Thompson but has since become characteristic of all Phoenix Air. "We'll be ready."

For Dent it wasn't just his vacation that'd ended but any peace at all for the foreseeable future. He spent that weekend clearing the decks, and early on Monday morning he headed straight to the office. First thing he did was google what he'd just gotten himself into. News out of West Africa was bleak. An outbreak spreading across three countries, casualties skyrocketing, hospitals closing, panic and violence and bodies in the street. Even for a guy who'd spent the previous two decades getting planes into and out of dangerous places, the situation was scary. He called Walters. The two Americans, a doctor and a medical aid, were stuck in Liberia but otherwise, Walters told him, details were scarce. Dent did more googling, more thinking. He called back. Kept calling. Each time a new question popped into his head he grabbed the phone.

Sometime around midmorning Dent called to ask who was actually in charge of this mission, and the answer, essentially, was *you are*. For months Samaritan's Purse had asked for help containing the outbreak, warning anyone who would listen that it could spread beyond the region, beyond Africa. But Washington had never warmed to the fight or developed a plan, and so when this particular crisis arose the US government was caught flat-footed. This was exactly the sort of problem Operational Medicine was created to handle, but obtaining the necessary clearances for the State Department to get *involved* involved, officially, would take too long. Walters could serve as facilitator, but the task of crossing an ocean and wandering into a country gone mad with hemorrhagic fever to bring people home quickly and safely would fall entirely on Phoenix.

As a guy who keeps his anxiety in check through planning, what Dent wanted more than anything was information. And he got it that afternoon. Shortly after lunch the phone rang again. It was Ken Isaacs at the Samaritan's Purse command center. In the background Dent could hear voices and commotion, a rolling sea of fear and frustration but also, for the first time in days, hope. But hope was on the clock. Isaacs jumped right in: "If you can do this, how's it going to work?"

Phoenix's biocontainment unit could hold only one patient, so they'd have to make two trips. The destination was the Serious Communicable Diseases Unit at Atlanta's Emory University Hospital, chosen not only for its proximity to Phoenix Air but also because it sits just feet from the front door of the CDC. This would shorten the turnaround time back to Africa, but after factoring in decon and reequipping of the plane, plus mandatory crew rest, there'd still be a couple days between flights. That meant a very difficult decision would have to be made in Monrovia about who got rescued and who waited, but that was for later. First they needed to come to terms.

Under sane conditions "coming to terms" would mean lawyers and contracts, a back-and-forth negotiation for revision and approval. But these were lunatic days and the two people in Monrovia couldn't wait that long. They were already three days into an eight-day survival window. This needed to happen now, and so it needed to happen with nothing more legally binding than a promise that when this whole thing was over, Samaritan's Purse wouldn't run out on the bill. Dent chewed on this for a minute. If it seemed each new development left Phoenix more exposed than the last, that's because it did. He sat quietly thinking through the myriad ways this could go wrong, how the company he and his brother had built could fall apart, and all the while he could hear people on the other end of the line, gathered around Isaacs and listening, hoping, some of them begging, saying *Please make this happen.* "This" being Dent agreeing to organize two flights into Monrovia and repatriating a pair of Americans with experimental technology that might or might not protect his people from the scariest death imaginable, and doing the whole thing on a handshake deal made over the telephone. That right there is about as Phoenix as it gets.

A deep breath and Dent said, "Okay. We'll do it."

15

Cartersville is a town of twenty-three thousand people just forty miles north of Atlanta. Home of the world's first outdoor Coca-Cola sign, of a nineteenth-century Baptist missionary who survived the Boxer Rebellion in China, and also of Rebecca Ann Felton—enthusiastic supporter of lynching and the first woman to serve (for one day) in the United States Senate. It has a historic downtown, an old courthouse, ancient Native American burial mounds, and at least one intersection dominated by a Buc-ee's convenience store and gas station. Big homes, quaint homes, mobile homes, they all gaze toward a treetop horizon interrupted only by Kennesaw Mountain and the cooling towers of a coal-fired power plant. It's a land of hay fields, red clay, and cicadas, of country two-lanes forever haunted by armadillos dead and liquifying on the shoulder. Cartersville is less than an hour from the South's largest city but is, by any measure, a world away.

It's also where Phoenix Air is headquartered. The campus sprawls across a massive stretch of open land and is divided in two by a narrow road that rises and falls as it reaches out over the rolling fields. On the east side is a small airfield and runway, a half-dozen hangars, a control tower, and a welcome center that sells Phoenix Air golf shirts. To the west is their two-story headquarters, a building known to everyone who doesn't work inside it as the Silver Palace. Dent got to headquarters early on Tuesday morning and stood outside waiting with Dr. Mike. They were joined shortly by Doug Olson, a forty-two-year-old doctor from California who moved to Georgia for his medical residency and never left. He was now ER director for a local hospital and had been flying missions with Phoenix since 2006. When Doug first heard about Brantly and Writebol he figured Phoenix might somehow be involved in bringing them home. It wasn't an hour later that Dr. Mike called.

"Let me guess," Doug said. "This is about Ebola."

Between the three of them, there was experience to burn. But standing around, waiting for the circus to arrive, they were uneasy. They'd never been through a demonstration quite this elaborate before. Walters told them he was bringing the world to their doorstep, but exactly what that meant and how it would go had not been made entirely clear. They stood talking, waiting, occasionally glancing down the road through the shimmer of heat waves hovering just above the asphalt. At 10 a.m. the first car appeared in the distance.

They arrived separately and at different times, and kicked off an avalanche of handshakes and introductions, of government agencies listed in lieu of backstory. *Hi, I'm from the State Department. I'm from the CDC. From the DOD. From USAMRIID.* Half the agencies Dent hadn't heard of. When the last hand had been shaken, he nodded to Walters and said, "All right, let's go over to the east side."

On the far side of the airstrip lie the hangars where Phoenix's mechanics and machinists maintain and modify the company's aircraft. These are massive metal buildings, loud with activity and hot from the sun. The biocontainment unit had been set up in one of them, and when Dent got in that morning he had everybody clear out so the place would be quiet. There was nothing he could do about the heat. They stepped inside and were dwarfed by the scale of the hangar, by the flat-gray Gulfstream III Gray Bird parked dead center. Off to the side and tiny in relation to everything else, sat the reason they were all here, the biocontainment system—a clear plastic tent supported by a twelve-by-five aluminum frame and connected by hoses, tubes, and wires to a filtration system and a handful of medical devices. It looked too small and simple, maybe even too fragile, for the task they'd come to consider. The experts walked around it, they stooped to look inside, they asked questions. Medical questions. Questions about training and its practical application in the jet. Dr. Mike, Doug, and Vance demonstrated the features, explained their policies and procedures, and led them into the Gray Bird so they could see how it was integrated into the aircraft.

Dent stood listening, sweating. The medical jargon was over his head, spoken between doctors and scientists, and there wasn't much for him to say. His mind started to wander. The tent was revolutionary—small enough to fit into a jet, big enough for treating a patient—and nothing like it existed anywhere else in the world. He wondered if they understood what they were seeing and all that had gone into it, that this unassuming tent was actually a highly advanced, if wholly unproven, piece of biocontainment technology that Phoenix had whipped up a few years prior. *Whipped up* in the sense that the engineers in the movie *Apollo 13* whipped up a work-around for Tom Hanks when he was a quarter-million miles away and circling the moon in a broken spaceship. Meaning Phoenix Air had willed it into being with ingenuity and determination and the specific sort of desperation that's required to save lives under impossible conditions.

16

It began in 2007 when the CDC summoned Dent without explanation to their Atlanta headquarters. Dent didn't know who or what he might need, so he grabbed Dr. Mike and Rickey Smith, an experienced test pilot and aircraft engineer, and together they drove down. The CDC borders the campus of Emory University, a private college and associated hospital tucked into a neighborhood of towering oaks and stately homes, meaning students, professors, and doctors all mingle with some of the world's scariest known pathogens. The facility doesn't look like much from the street, just a guarded front gate blocking a narrow drive that slopes down toward a crowded huddle of buildings. Dent, Dr. Mike, and Rickey were waved through and ushered to a dimly lit room full of TV screens that flashed a bewildering array of data. It dawned on them that this was it, the CDC's crisis center, a sort of war room where the agency monitors incidents and outbreaks around the world. This was privileged space. The nerve center. After a few minutes, the agency's chief operating officer entered, along with their top doctor and a handful of infectious disease experts. Together they laid out the problem before them.

As part of the international response to infectious disease, the CDC's special investigative teams deploy to emerging hot spots around the world. They'd done it in the past for outbreaks of cholera and more recently for sudden acute respiratory syndrome, a terrifying airborne virus with the potential to kill millions. SARS had appeared from nowhere in 2003, then quietly slipped away. Everyone agreed after it was gone and hadn't wiped us all out that we'd dodged a bullet. But SARS periodically returned, as did bird flu, swine flu, and others. There'd always be some new variety of contagious death on the horizon. The CDC's doctors were routinely deployed around the world to deal with them, and it was critical that they continue to do so.

"But we're having trouble getting our doctors to respond."

Dent asked why, and here the CDC officials exchanged nervous glances. The problem boiled down to a policy called treat-in-place, which says that if you send an infectious disease specialist to China or Vietnam or North Africa—anywhere dangerous viruses are on the move—and she gets sick, then she stays right there. Medicine, staff, whatever's needed, can be sent to her but she won't be released from quarantine and allowed to go home until she's virus-free. Or dead. With the world more interconnected every day the pace of these deployments was increasing, but no provision had been made for evacuating staff should they get sick. This was becoming an issue. Families didn't want them to go and hesitation had grown among the doctors themselves. The obvious solution was for the CDC to guarantee any stricken staff member an immediate flight home with expert care, but less obvious was how they'd make that happen. Enter Phoenix.

Here the tone of the meeting shifted and sort of shook loose into an informal conversation that wound its way around possibilities and technicalities, all of them hypothetical. High-level spitballing, basically. Theoretical. Rickey Smith began to tune out. He became an airplane mechanic and engineer out of necessity—if you lived in Gadsden, Alabama in the 1960s and wanted to fly, you either learned to fix your own plane or else you stayed on the ground. This ethos stuck, and as talk floated around him, Rickey grabbed a pad of paper and quietly—he doesn't say much to begin with—began sketching. Rickey's a big guy, almost hulking, with a glowering expression. His voice is gravelly and deep Alabama and used only after careful deliberation. As the experts talked logistical hurdles and technical difficulties, Rickey decided the problem wasn't all that complex. Really, you just needed an airtight enclosure and the ability to create a negative pressure environment, which you do by making the air pressure inside the enclosure lower than it is in the cabin so that air is sucked in but cannot get out. He'd already worked with positive pressure and figured you could do one just as easy as the other. So check that off the list.

Then Rickey turned his attention to the frame. This was a little trickier because it had to be all things at once—big enough inside to allow room for patient care, but small enough to fit in a jet and sturdy enough to survive a crash, but also light enough to be mobile. He circled the problem several times before an idea struck. The week before, Rickey and his wife had been on vacation in Florida, and she'd brought along a beach tent that hung from its frame by loops sewn onto the outside of the fabric. Basically, the frame was an exoskeleton that didn't clutter the inside at all. The talking continued as Rickey did a little math, tallied the inner dimensions of the Gulfstream III, and figured out how big an exoskeleton he could get away with. Then he sketched out the general outlines of the tent, putting a vacuum pump up front to draw air and an exhaust valve in back. They'd need a filtration system, but anything that would fit on a plane, work with their tent, and also make deadly air safe to breathe probably didn't exist and would have to be made in house. He'd worry about that later.

Within a few minutes he had the basic idea sketched out. He then excused himself from the table and called his engineering team back at Phoenix. He had his sketch pad and he walked them through the whole thing, modifying and shifting as he went, then asked, "Y'all know any reason we can't do this?" The engineers in Cartersville all shook their heads and said no. Nobody could see why this couldn't be done.

Rickey went back to the table—they were still talking—and casually told Dent he could do it, that more or less he already knew how. Simple as that. Dent nodded and leaned back in his seat. Of all the emotions he was feeling in that moment, surprise was not among them. What Phoenix does maybe better than anyone is find people, oftentimes people everyone else has overlooked, people with ingenuity and competence and self-reliance, with a willingness to serve and a dash of Mark's *hell-yeah-I'll-do-that* persona, and then set them loose to do whatever it is they do best. They come alive in that freedom and their unfurling is what conjures the strange magic of Phoenix Air. In this nuanced, almost elusive recipe Dent is the unnamable ingredient that completes the circuit and brings it all to life. He's an organizer, a facilitator, a showman. His sense of flair is extravagant—the man married a debutant named

Pepper—and in the drama of the moment, sitting in the CDC war room, screens flashing danger, experts predicting a perilous future and inviting him along for the ride, Dent got inspired. He got expansive.

"When I was a kid John Kennedy said that with enough money and enough time we'll go to the moon." He looked around. "Give us a little of the same and we'll make anything happen."

A loud *riiiiiiiip* echoed as a long section of duct tape was yanked from a fat white roll. It was a few weeks later and the Phoenix team watched as an engineer carefully laid out the tent's dimensions on the hangar floor. When he was done, they stood looking at it—a twelve-by-five rectangle that felt, when you stood inside it, like little more than a coffin. And that was before you considered that nearly a third of it had to be reserved for an antechamber where providers could remove dirty PPE before exiting. That left just eight feet for the patient compartment. Eight feet for the bed, for the medical supplies, for the monitors and IV pumps and ventilators. Eight feet for two people, one of them working and the other slowly dying. This didn't feel to Dr. Mike like enough room but there it was, undeniable and stark as a chalk outline on the floor of a crime scene.

Chris Allen, meanwhile, was in the break room with a cup of coffee and a pencil, sketching on a napkin. Not long after the meeting at the CDC, specs for a filter had been sent to an engineering firm and the drawings had just arrived. Chris had a complicated relationship with engineers. He considered them highly educated, maybe overeducated, and in his opinion they've never met a project they couldn't overengineer. Chris worshiped at the altar of simplicity. He grew up on a south Georgia farm where he learned welding, electrical, engine repair, and also that the system least likely to fail was often the simplest. He left home to become an airplane mechanic, got airframe and powerplant (A&P) certified—a long and grueling process of apprenticeships and written exams with dizzying fail rates—and then spent a couple decades at Delta before accepting a job at Phoenix. The task of making, assembling, and installing the filter had fallen to Chris. He flipped through the drawings again then called in Tobin Jenkins. Like Chris, Tobin's an A&P mechanic, but all similarities stop there. Where Chris is short with a soft voice, Tobin is tall with a great big smile and personality to match. Tobin looked at the drawings and got to thinking the same thing Chris was thinking—overengineered. Then they got to work.

Chris had already built one filter according to the engineering specs and was unsurprised to find that it leaked. Industry standard allowed for a tiny amount of leakage, but it would be his coworkers in that jet, so only a zero-leak filter would do. So he and Tobin redesigned it. Then they redesigned their redesign. Most of the problems seemed to stem from the welds, so they machined a filter from a solid piece of aluminum. They changed gasket material, altered the size and weight, simplified and then simplified again. Each redesign started with Chris and Tobin in the break room, scribbling specs on a napkin and then carrying them to the machinists who churned out yet another prototype. Eventually they got there. A zero-leak filter that integrated with the tent and weighed in at 120 pounds fully assembled.

Meanwhile, Rickey was hard at work reversing the Gray Bird's airflow. Normally, fresh air enters a plane through the fuselage and circulates back to front, where it exits through an exhaust valve beneath the pilot's seat. So, if there was a failure in the containment system—a rip in the tent wall, sudden depressurization, loss of power—contaminated air would move toward the cockpit and concentrate directly beneath the pilots. Blowing smallpox or SARS, or really any pathogen, directly onto your pilots midflight isn't ideal. To fix it, Rickey modified the jet itself so that when the containment system was in use air flowed not toward the exhaust valve up front but to one that

Chris fabricated to fit on the back. What made this so tricky, essentially, was pressurization. The interior of a plane is pressurized so the passengers and crew can breathe as the plane gains altitude. If the plane were to over-pressurize, it'd start blowing out rivets and the exterior would split open, and if that happened at forty thousand feet you'd be in trouble. It's the release valve that keeps this from happening, so if you're going to reverse the airflow by cutting off one release valve and creating another, you better make sure you get it right.

Once everything was ready and they had a prototype of the full containment system built and installed in one of the modified Gray Birds, Rickey and Dr. Mike flew up to the federal proving grounds in Maryland for test flights. The DOD, CDC, FAA, they all wanted assurance that not only would the system work under normal conditions, but that it wouldn't kill everyone on board if something went wrong. The government also needed proof that the modifications to reverse the airflow were safe and functioned properly. The tent was placed on a shake table and brutalized in every conceivable manner to see if it could withstand the force of a crash (it could), and it was then loaded back onto the Gray Bird for test flights. The general pattern for these was simple—Rickey would climb to forty-five thousand feet, dump cabin pressure, and then rocket back to Earth in an emergency decent.

Dr. Mike, buckled into the back and wearing an oxygen mask, monitored the tent to see if it leaked or was compromised in any way.

In a test flight you're intentionally pushing an aircraft over the outer edge of its limits just to see how it behaves. The risks are obvious but tempered with planning—if you fully understand what it is you're testing for, then you should also know what failure looks like and be able to recognize its signs before disaster strikes. But the people who volunteer to pilot those flights, the ones that may end in *failure* and *disaster*, would never use those words. A test pilot at the controls of an airplane gone haywire and torpedoing to Earth would, by contrast, say the aircraft diverged from its predicted parameters. Rickey had plenty of aircraft warn him they were about to become unpredictable but sometimes, early in his career, he missed the signs. One time his plane stalled, pitched, and then rolled all the way over. Dangling upside down and about to crash is maybe the wrong time to realize an aircraft won't be passing the test. But if you're wired a certain kind of way, each near-disaster becomes a lesson in itself. And over a lifetime those lessons build to an understanding that more closely resembles instinct than knowledge. All of Rickey's instincts came to bear in creating the containment system, which, as expected, passed the tests.

The various branches of government involved in the project then reviewed the data and signed off on use of the tent. It now even had an official name: the Aeromedical Biological Containment System or ABCS. This part of the process took the longest, a couple years in all. There's red tape and there's more red tape—and then there's the FAA. In that time, several pressing outbreaks had run their respective bell curves and things quieted down. The dozen or so ABCS units already manufactured were packed into bundles and placed on a shelf.

Passing by the storage unit one day in late 2013, Dr. Mike looked at Vance and said, "Sure hope we never have to use these things."

And now here they were in July 2014 considering whether or not to do just that. Dent didn't think the moment of decision ought to be somber, nor did he want it to be rushed. They should enter into this as clear-eyed as possible, and it's hard to think clearly when you're half-melted in a sunbaked hangar. He stepped out in front of Walters and the scientists and held up his hand.

"What do you say we sit down in the AC and talk about it?"

17

The second floor of the Silver Palace is the nexus of Phoenix. Mark's office, Dent's office. Their lawyer. A dispatch area surrounded by screens, phones, and two-way radios. The group filed past all the activity without a sound and took seats at the four round tables in the breakroom. Dent made sure everyone had water, and for a few minutes they just talked. Nothing serious, nothing about the tent or Ebola, just people getting to know each other, relieved to have escaped the heat. Dent looked at the government experts, about a dozen in all, and still couldn't tell who was who or which one was most important. Hard to say if it even mattered. He took a seat, twisted open his water bottle. Drank. The guy sitting next to him had his cell sitting out on the table. He'd been attached to it all morning, flipping it on then off, checking it, rechecking it, obsessively, like a teenager. Now the phone started ringing. He very quickly reached for it.

"Yes, Mr. President."

Dent stopped mid-swallow. Almost choked but tried to play it cool. He turned his head a little, eyebrows slowly raising.

"Yes sir, we're about to make a decision." Pause. "I'll let you know, sir."

Then he hung up. Dent felt his throat go dry.

"Was that Obama?"

The man nodded. "Yeah, he's very interested in what's about to happen."

Maybe the AC wasn't working because Dent was hot again, and he finished off his water thinking, *No pressure, we got this, no pressure at all*, the whole room swelling with the low-grade hum of idle conversation like all this was normal, the kind of thing you just do on a Tuesday morning while the President of the United States waits for your decision. Dent scanned the room to find Walters, who hadn't said much up to now, then nodded to him and said, "All right, how do you want to do this?"

Walters's primary concern that morning was finding a way to rescue two Americans who'd volunteered to help strangers and now needed to be saved themselves. But something else, something even larger and unspoken, hung in the balance. The people dying of Ebola in Sierra Leone, Guinea, and Liberia needed effective treatment to survive, but nearly every hospital in the region had already been overrun and now existed—*if* they existed—in name only. It wasn't possible to evacuate every diagnosed patient out of the hot zone and into a city with a functioning healthcare system, and so the key, Walters believed, was bringing critical care to them. They needed medicine and medical supplies, but above all they needed medical professionals, people like Kent Brantly and Nancy Writebol, who were willing to face the risks and deliver care.

And from the very beginning these professionals had answered the call. The world's governments might've been slow to respond to Ebola, but its individual experts leapt in. Doctors, nurses, and epidemiologists, many of them from across Africa, but also from Europe and the US, had volunteered to fight the outbreak—and now Ebola was the leading cause of death among them. Just like the two diagnoses had a chilling effect on the staff at ELWA, the mounting casualties had begun to scare off these desperately needed volunteers. Both the WHO and MSF, the two largest organizations in the fight, were having trouble recruiting doctors to work in the hot zone. Those who did go often returned home stressed, exhausted, and full of horror stories. Their families pressured them not to return.

It's what the CDC had feared back in 2007 when the idea for the ABCS first emerged, only now those fears had come to life. At the very moment a deadly outbreak was threatening to spill over its regional borders and spread to who knows where, the people most capable of stopping it had become hesitant to go where they were needed because the risks had simply become too great. Those still willing to go had done the math and accepted the risk but still wanted, if something went wrong, the promise of dying at home. For that reason, this rescue mission had implications that extended beyond the lives of Kent and Nancy. It was about protecting the international force of experts who protected the rest of us. There were plenty of people who wanted to help in West Africa. But no one wanted to die there. What they needed in return for their service was the same thing they'd be volunteering to provide—hope. Phoenix Air, the ABCS, all eighteen people seated in this room and about to pass judgement, that's exactly what they'd be delivering. Hope.

Walters stood and looked around the room. Then he asked the government experts if the system would work. They all agreed the ABCS was exactly what they'd been looking for. This system would work. Dr. Mike looked around the room thinking, *Holy shit, this is gonna happen*. He was confident that the ABCS would do what it had been designed to do. But it's one thing to believe the system was safe and another thing altogether to promise your coworkers that it's safe enough for them to bet their lives on. And as the guy making the decision of whether or not they could pull off this mission, that's exactly what Dr. Mike would be doing.

"Okay," Walters said. "How many people think this is appropriate? Raise your hand?"

The government experts all raised their hands. Then came the sound of shifting chairs as they looked around to see if anyone disagreed. Vance leaned over to Dr. Mike and whispered, "That's because they're not gonna be in this thing. You and I are."

Now Walters turned to the guys from Phoenix. Like everyone else here he believed the ABCS would work, which meant the only remaining question was if, when the time came, they'd have the nerve to spend twelve hours locked inside an aircraft with a terrifying pathogen. Walters is accomplished and educated and highly regarded, both connected and action-oriented, but also very wry. "Guys, you'll be the ones in the cylindrical death tube. Can you do it or not?"

Here, Dent said nothing. This was a decision for the medical people. However much you believed in the system, Ebola was not particularly well understood and the risks were very real. Everyone who went would be a volunteer, which he judged to be a very personal decision. First to respond was Doug Olson.

Doug was younger than Vance and Dr. Mike, newer to the profession, newer to Phoenix, but every bit as accustomed to danger. He started working in operational and tactical medicine back in California where he rode along with gang units in San Bernardino. During his med school residency he went through SWAT school, and then ran ground and helicopter missions with the Columbia County Sheriff's Department in southwest Georgia. That led to work with the DEA and the ATF and eventually with the FBI, who wanted a tactical medical component to accompany their hostage rescue and rapid response teams. He had a strong desire to serve, and he often described himself as having an abnormally low response to danger.

Doug didn't blink, just nodded yes, he could do it. Vance was next, but he had reservations. They'd trained in the ABCS, but not for Ebola. They didn't have protocols for using PPE, and come to think of it he wasn't certain they even had PPE. He didn't know what to expect, and that made him anxious. But Vance was extremely experienced and knowledgeable, so much so that he could be intimidating to work with. He trusted the ABCS and his coworkers, he trusted himself. With some time and practice, he figured, they could whip themselves into shape and so he, too, said yes. Then Vance, along with everyone else, turned to Dr. Mike, the medical director.

Dr. Mike was nervous. He didn't know how Kent and Nancy had gotten the virus, but he assumed that if his team protected themselves they'd be safe. Tricky time to assume anything—who knows what they might run into during the transports—but at some point they'd have to trust their equipment, process, and experience to carry them through. And anyway, it was missions like this they'd signed on for, the impossible. He nodded at Walters.

"Yeah," he said. "We'll do it."

The man with the phone immediately jumped up and was out the door—*Yessir, Mr. President, the system can be used*. The other experts filed out behind him, Walters saying he'd be in touch about timeline and clearances, Dent nodding but not really listening, his mind churning through the million details that lay ahead. Vance and Doug went across the street to begin searching up protocols and PPE. Dr. Mike, carrying the weight of responsibility, was last to leave. Ebola is often referred to as the caregiver's disease because healthcare workers are stricken and killed by it in disproportionate numbers. As the one who said it was safe, if anyone got sick it would be on him.

18

Jonathan Jackson stood over on the east side of the airfield, sweating in a blue Phoenix Air flight suit. He watched the line of rental cars drive off with a sinking feeling in his guts, like events beyond his control were taking shape and gaining speed. Like the momentum might carry him away and there wasn't much he could do about it. Whatever was happening had first hit his radar two days before, during a layover in Anchorage. He was on his way back from Tianjin, China, coming off the type of long medical flight that kept him out of the country and on the move for 200 days a year. It was eight or nine in the morning and Jonathan was sitting in a hotel bar when Dr. Mike called to say, "As soon as you get back to Cartersville, come see me." Which felt strange. He was an ICU nurse, had been at Phoenix for a while now, and it wasn't normal for Dr. Mike to reach out before he even made it home to say, "Don't go home." The television behind the bar was going on about the Ebola outbreak and how among the dying were two Americans whose families wanted them back, and right then he knew. Jonathan took a long swallow of beer and said to the pilot sitting next to him, "Shit, I guess that's what this is all about."

And now the sight of government experts driving away pretty much confirmed his suspicions. Behind him a plane took off and he squinted to watch it disappear into the sun. Jonathan grew up in a North Georgia town of 4,800 people and was making nothing but bad decisions when he stopped long enough to take stock of his life. He was headed nowhere good and decided instead to follow his mother and brother into nursing. He bounced around a couple different hospitals, worked trauma for a while at Erlanger Hospital in Tennessee, got burned out, and was looking for a change. He was thirty-three when he met Vance and now, a decade later, he was still at Phoenix. Jonathan was a big guy, country, and when asked to go very bad places to deal with scary things his reaction tended to be something along the lines of *What time are we wheels up*? Multisystem trauma, rare diseases, fragile ICU patients, the half-dead, mostly dead, sure-to-be-dead, even people who were only vaguely ill but hit misfortune in places so hairy you keep the engines running on the tarmac—he'd dealt with all that and more, usually in the cramped fuselage of an aging Gulfstream. But Ebola was something else. Ten minutes ago, if someone had asked him to describe himself or his coworkers, he'd have said, *Hell, we can do anything.* But now, watching those cars pull away with reality starting to hit, the thing going through his mind was *I think I gotta talk to my wife.*

There's a flag nailed to the wall of the medical hangar at Phoenix. It's blazing orange and in the center is a large caduceus—the winged staff with two entwined snakes that's become an international symbol for doctor. Circling the caduceus in large black letters are two sentences. *No one is coming. It's up to us.* It's doubtful any slogan could better sum up the situation Phoenix's med staff found themselves in. When Jonathan reached the medical hangar, Dr. Mike, Doug Olson, and Vance Ferebee were already there. They laid the whole thing out for him, including the call to the president, and then got down to work. The nature of Ebola dictated that they'd have to move fast or there'd be no point in moving at all—at best, they probably had two days to prepare. By informal consent they decided Dr. Mike would stay in Atlanta to coordinate the effort, which meant Doug would be the doctor on both flights, with Vance and Jonathan as the two nurses. Unlike hospital medicine with its rigid hierarchies, flight medicine is loose and egalitarian. There's no backup in a plane, pretty much no anything. Your only resources are whatever people and gear you can cram into the aircraft, and to get the most out of everyone, all are given an equal voice. Jonathan was only just now joining this particular circus, but he sat down and began doing his part to chip away at the problem—how often any one of them would be in the tent with the patient, how long they'd stay, how they'd exit safely. Ultimately, these were the sort of things they'd hammer out together. But moving past the hysteria and coming to grips with the fear of being locked in a plane with Ebola, each of them had to sort that out alone.

Phoenix Air had never done a mission quite like this. They had no protocols to guide them, so Vance went online to see what he could find. Pretty much what he found was nothing. Both the WHO and MSF had posted rudimentary guidelines, but none of them applied to treating highly infectious diseases at forty thousand feet. The WHO, for instance, called for the construction of a large decon chamber and then spraying everyone down, head-to-toe, with a bleach solution each time they exited the treatment area. Fine for a hospital but totally impossible in an airplane. Jonathan looked at Vance, who shrugged and then turned off his computer and announced to the room, "Guess we'll have to make our own manual."

Next came PPE. Again, the medical community

had differing views on what was adequate, and none of them accounted for the difficulties of outfitting a skeleton crew at work in a confined space. They'd have to improvise and started jotting down ideas on a pad of paper. One full-body Tyvek suit. One plastic gown, worn over the suit. One N95 face mask. One pair of goggles. Two pairs of gloves—the outer pair pulled up over the sleeves of the suit to protect the wrists. One hood to cover their heads and two pairs of surgical booties over their shoes. So now they knew what was needed, but here another problem arose—they didn't have it. Or at least nowhere near enough of it. Vance volunteered to go to the store and buy as much PPE as he could find. But because there aren't biohazard stores on every corner selling gear for the apocalypse, he wound up buying everything they'd wear to protect themselves against Ebola from Home Depot. In the meantime, he suggested everyone go home and get their affairs in order. From here on out there wouldn't be much rest.

Jonathan drove a couple hours north to his house in Ringgold, Georgia, where he showered and unpacked his bag from the Tianjin trip, which was now a lifetime ago. He no longer told his family all the sordid details of where he was going and what for—it wasn't always helpful for them to know what he was dealing with—but this was different. He walked into the kitchen to find his wife, Joanne, and two of their three daughters sitting at the table. His oldest child was out of the house, but the younger two, in eighth and tenth grade at the time, were waiting when he got there. Jonathan sat down and, in as matter-of-fact a way as he could, explained the situation. Joanne said nothing, just leaned back and let the girls work their way through it. They were quiet for a second and then got loud. They didn't like this and didn't want him to do it. Didn't think he should go, period, that he should refuse. The girls talked their way around it until eventually his middle daughter, Maddie, got quiet. She dug a fingernail into the table.

"This is your job," she said, looking up at him. "This could be you stuck in another country, dying, and somebody could have to go get you, so . . ." she trailed off, shrugged, circled back. "It's not fair for us to stop you from getting someone else."

There was a little more talking and some hugging, then the girls left. Jonathan looked up at Joanne, who hadn't said anything up to this point. There were so many times he'd gone off to dangerous places, so many times he was supposed to be home in three days but returned in seven. She'd gotten as used to it as best she could, but it was never easy.

"Just trust your gut," she told him. "If your gut says don't go, don't go."

19

Linda Mobula felt her insides tighten then convulse. She lurched forward and vomited blood all over the room. She was feverish and clammy, shivering so hard her bones ached. She was dying, liquifying, she knew it; there was no stopping it and—. She woke with a start. Sat up in bed. Looked around. Just another nightmare.

This had become her reality. To wake up hot and trembling, her whole body covered in sweat. She fumbled on the nightstand for the thermometer and took her temperature. Normal. Impossible. She took it again. Fell back in the sheets. The rational part of her brain knew she'd only had a nightmare, again, that being surrounded by the sick and dying, that treating Kent—who she saw as an almost perfect reflection of herself—had gotten to her, was wearing her down. Wearing them all down. She knew these things but it didn't stop the voice of fear from whispering things she wanted to forget. Like how she shared PPE with a

Liberian nurse who had since gotten sick or how, in an uncharacteristic moment of carelessness, she'd nearly torn her glove while treating Kent. The virus was all around them; it was everywhere and her colleagues were falling, and no matter how rational she tried to be she couldn't help but wonder who was next. Linda lay there a few moments, breathing, just long enough to let reason take control. To relax. Then she rolled over and reached for the thermometer.

By sunup she was getting texts from Kent, and they didn't stop. At her house, at the Ebola treatment center, at a staff meeting, her phone would *ping* with another message—

I'm worried about my electrolytes.

Ping!

The IV bag's running low.

Ping!

Just want to make sure I have enough potassium.

Ping!

Is it time for another round of antibiotics?

Doctors are the worst patients. She'd text back that she was in charge and he should let her make the decisions, but the texts continued. They were constant, almost comical, but at the same time understandable. Ebola patients are separated for treatment and then isolated in their separation—no one comes near them without gloves and masks; no one touches them. When

Kent was working in the ETC he'd gone out of his way to break through that crushing loneliness, and now the isolation was his. Amber and the kids were back in the States and the people who lived in the other half of his duplex had been forced out after his diagnosis—they were only given a few minutes to leave and most of their belongings were burned. If he needed help, it could take as long as two hours for Linda or Lance to get there, suit up, and go in. The sickness, plus the otherness, was beginning to cause confusion. He'd wake up anxious, convinced someone was in his house, and call out, "Who's there?! Is anybody in here?"

Linda made her way to Kent's house, suited up outside then went in. She was never certain what to expect when she got there. Ebola is a roller coaster of dips and crests, and Kent's symptoms had become concerning. He had blood in his stool and had also begun vomiting blood. The whites of his eyes were red and he was covered in the telltale Ebola rash that results from blood vessels bursting beneath the skin. These were ominous signs. Signs that his chances of survival were dropping and that maybe it was death he'd heard lurking in the dim corners of his house. Linda recognized all this, but then of course so did Kent. It was one thing to treat a patient who was dying and another altogether to treat a patient who understood that fact.

When she got to his room Kent was in bed. He said

he felt a little better today, but even this was mixed news. They'd both witnessed a phenomenon called pseudo-remission, where a patient suddenly and inexplicably improves before crashing and then dying. Was he *actually* feeling better or was this the calm before the storm? Linda hung a new IV bag to replenish the electrolytes he'd lost due to the bleeding and sweating and vomiting, to the diarrhea—it was horrifying, this disease, and humiliating. Next, she pushed one dose each of antibiotics and antimalarials. Neither of these drugs had been studied enough in Ebola patients to fully understand what they did or how, but they seemed to help and that was enough. Finally, she gave him morphine for the pain.

Given the circumstances, that was all she could do. All they did for anyone. There were no labs, and so as helpful as it would've been to take blood for a workup, there was no point. Nor did they do any diagnostics. She'd never even taken his blood pressure—that would just contaminate the equipment and they didn't have enough to go around. But she could be there. Kent couldn't see her face, but he heard her voice and derived whatever comfort he could from her presence. It wasn't high-tech Western medicine but it was powerful, and anyway it was all she had. Linda felt compassion for all her patients but Kent was a fellow doctor. She wasn't married yet, didn't have a family, but she hoped for one and sitting there listening to Kent take calls from home, hearing his kids sing to him over FaceTime, she couldn't help but wonder. About how all this would turn out for Kent, about whether his kids would have to go on without their father and Amber without her husband, and though she tried to push it aside or down or away, Linda couldn't help but wonder if something went wrong and Kent died, would it turn out to have been her fault.

20

Dent got out of bed Wednesday morning having barely slept at all. He dressed, jumped in his car, and swung out of the circular driveway in front of his Buckhead home for the thirty-minute drive to Cartersville. That Phoenix represented simultaneously the safest and only hope of bringing two sick Americans home was now a clear and established fact, as was their willingness, as Walters put it, to step inside the cylindrical tube of death. Scientists from a dozen federal agencies had signed off on the plan. The president himself had given the operation his tacit approval. But the reality of bringing Kent and Nancy back would require the cooperation of the dozens of federal agencies with jurisdiction over the nation's health and security, over its borders, airports, and highways. This meant making them comfortable with Phoenix Air, a company most of them had never heard of, and its audacious plan—which of course was to import Ebola into the United States. TSA, Homeland Security, FAA, Department of

Defense, Customs, nobody from these agencies knew anything about Ebola other than to fear it. They may as well have been discussing the Black Plague. Once word of the operation got out, these agencies would unleash a tsunami of objections, all of which Dent had to calmly counter with simple but foolproof plans.

Upon arriving at the Silver Palace, Dent, together with Walters, presided over a series of marathon conference calls, each with thirty or more high-ranking officials from every imaginable federal agency. Walters would kick things off and then turn it over to Dent who'd detail Phoenix Air's experience and capabilities, the life and death stakes of the operation, its moving parts, and exactly how it would all come together. Somewhere in the middle of all this a voice would cut in over the line:

Hey guys, TSA here and what I'm wondering is...

And just like that the conversation would be hijacked. Ultimately, what the TSA rep wanted to know was how many of their agency's regulations would be violated and how often. And the TSA wasn't alone. Even the health agencies—CDC, Health and Human Services—had serious questions. On call after call, they fired their concerns at Dent, who found himself explaining and promising and flat-out tap dancing like never before in his life.

How do you intend to show your passports? How do we

know who you say is on the plane is really on the plane? Where are you going to enter the US? How will you keep your medical staff from exposing your pilots and then your pilots from exposing the rest of us?

For the medical questions, he referred back to the ABCS, to their training, their protocols—which, technically, Vance was still trying to figure out. But why cloud the issue with too many details? As for the procedural concerns, Dent's answers were sometimes specific and others fired blindly, shotgun-style, always with a tinge of humor. "You don't have to collect paperwork on the ramp," Dent said. "We'll fax it to you ahead of time. For anything that needs to be communicated on the ground, we'll bring a little chalkboard along and hold it to the window. Your people won't ever come close to ours. And as for who's onboard—I guarantee there won't be any terrorists sneaking on there. *Nobody* wants to get on that plane."

A laugh over the line. A small but needed release. Then more questions. More work. We say *bureaucrat* like it's a dirty word, but the truth is the people on the other end of the line had dedicated themselves to protecting and serving the American public. It's a thankless job and, when done well, it's not the people doing the actual work but an elected official who gets the credit. But should there be a problem—and this mission was a rabbit warren of potential problems—the bureaucrats would be the ones hauled before Congress to explain why they allowed it to happen in the first place. It gradually became clear to Dent that they weren't saying *no* so much as *yeah, but*—the *but* coming in the form of a raft of legal and technical requirements so extensive that to follow them all was impossible. It was at this point, as the flow of conversation backed up and clogged, that Walters would step in. Among Walters's skills is the ability to distill a complicated problem to its essence. And when you got right down to it, the problem here was a combination of fear and inertia. Fear he could deal with—the medicine wasn't complicated, just misunderstood. Explain it, and the fear (mostly) goes away. Much more difficult was overcoming inertia. But for this, too, he had an answer. Step one: Reiterate the knowns. This is the problem; this is the plan. Keep it simple but direct. Step two: Determine what scares them the most. Respect and address their concerns. Step three: Adjust the plan and keep moving forward.

Walters believed everyone wanted to do the right thing; it's just that they also wanted this unconventional operation to adhere to their long-established conventions. It was impossible to do that, and anyway there wasn't time for it—the first patient would be landing in seventy-two hours; the clock was ticking. When people couldn't be swayed with reason, Walters would become what Dent liked to call the snowplow. He'd jump in over the chatter and say, "Look, this is an emergency situation and we're going to deal with it as best we can; you won't be blamed but you also won't stop it. This is happening."

21

Jonathan Jackson, Vance Ferebee, and Doug Olson stood in the hangar looking at all the gear Vance had bought the day before at Home Depot. Tyvek suits, plastic goggles, masks. Bundles and bundles of plastic sheeting. There was only one Gulfstream III modified for use with the ABCS, and everything hinged on that plane. Even a drop of partially digested blood vomited onto the Gray Bird's upholstered seats, which absolutely cannot be decontaminated, would leave the aircraft permanently Ebola positive and more or less knock them out of commission. To prevent it, they decided to drape every square inch of the interior in plastic anytime a patient was being loaded or unloaded. Vance wasn't sure which size would be too thick to tear but light enough to hang, so he bought nine-by-twelve sheets of plastic in various thicknesses, figuring they'd just test it out when the time came.

Now that they had all their PPE, it was time to

develop and then perfect procedures for getting into (donning) and out of (doffing) their gear. They'd never done this in the ABCS and certainly not under the life and death stakes of Ebola, but they all had experience with PPE. They were medical professionals. How hard could it be?

The first thing Jonathan noticed after climbing into his PPE was the heat. So much heat. The instant he put on the suit he began to sweat himself dry, could feel the energy drain down to his feet and out onto the floor. Best to get used to that now—however bad it was in Cartersville it wouldn't be any better in West Africa. It was also hard to see, hard to hear. Breathing was difficult and with two pairs of gloves on, forget about dexterity. He stepped inside the ABCS. The antechamber is a four-foot section at the front of the tent separated from both the treatment area and the outside world by a pair of doors that zip shut at either end. During the flights, they'd emerge from the treatment area, zip the door closed behind them, and then remove all PPE before unzipping the second door and stepping out of the ABCS. To remove gear, they'd start with the outer layers and methodically work their way in, pausing between various predesignated steps to decon their gloves. They developed a doffing process that included thirty steps and took about twenty minutes to complete. And they'd be doing all of it in an area not much bigger than a car trunk. Jonathan blinked as sweat ran into his eyes.

Aside from being narrow, the antechamber is only five feet tall. Jonathan stands about six feet and so he was doubled over at the waist, legs trembling before he even started. And this, the practice session, was as good as it was going to get. In flight the aircraft was liable to be climbing or descending or getting tossed around by turbulence. And there he'd be, crouching inside this tiny space for twenty minutes at a go, surrounded by Ebola and trying not to infect himself. He started working his way through the process—*disinfect the apron, then the outer gloves, remove both after checking for tears*—and almost immediately ran into trouble.

To remove the Tyvek suit, he was supposed to unzip the front and shrug his shoulders out, then roll the material down as he went so the whole thing was inside-out when he finally got it off. Imagine a banana peeling itself. But he couldn't get his shoulders out because the suit was too tight. And not just his suit, but all the suits. Vance had bought Tyvek suits that would fit them, but they discovered that the only way to wiggle out of the suit with enough ease that they didn't lose their balance and touch the side walls or the ceiling or some exposed bit of skin, was to be in a too-big suit. Probably two sizes too big. Comically big. So Vance went back to Home Depot. He got more Tyvek.

An hour later he returned with new suits, but all the old problems remained. Crouching in the antechamber, legs shaking, body wobbling, trying not to touch the sides or the ceiling, trying to balance on one foot while removing some item, they repeatedly lost their balance and touched something or dropped something or removed the PPE out of sequence and contaminated themselves. So far they were failing, and failure meant an accidental exposure to a highly infectious agent. Failure meant almost certain death for any or all of them. So they suited up and reimagined the entire process. Then did it again. And again. By noon the temperature was rising and everybody was hot and sweating, and tired from not sleeping the night before.

The general anxiety of wanting to get it right, the fear of messing it up, of Ebola, was all swirling around in their heads, mixing them up. So half the time they contaminated themselves and didn't know it, and the other half they only thought they did but couldn't be sure. It wasn't getting any better so they stopped and huddled to rethink the process. The problem was less the steps themselves than it was keeping the steps straight in their heads. What they needed was another pair of arms. Or at the very least another set of eyes. They decided to add a spotter. Now the person stepping out of the patient compartment and into the antechamber to doff wouldn't have to go through it alone. They'd have a buddy standing just outside the zipped door, calling out steps, warning if they were too close to the wall or the ceiling, letting them know they'd put a foot on the ground and now had to ditch the sock. The only thing that wasn't obvious about it was why they hadn't thought of it sooner.

Jonathan climbed back into his PPE and stepped into the patient chamber.

Vance stood outside the tent with a clipboard in his hand: "Okay, remove your outer booties."

Inside the tent, Jonathan removed his outer boot covers and then, when prompted, pulled off the outer gloves and stepped into the antechamber. With Vance calling out the steps, he disinfected his inner gloves and began the process of peeling himself out of the Tyvek suit. Right away he bumped his head on the roof and had to start over.

"Remove your outer booties."

He removed the boot covers, but he was hot and tired and rushing and he stepped into the antechamber with his outer gloves on and had to start over.

"Remove your outer booties."

This time he bumped the wall and had to start over.

"Remove your outer booties."

On and on. At one point he nearly made it through the entire twenty-minute process but was so delirious with heat and exhaustion that he reached up and wiped sweat from his eyes with a contaminated glove.

"You're dead," Vance said. "Start over."

"Try to do it facing us," Doug called. "Might help if you have eye contact."

The next time Jonathan touched his wrist. "Nope. You just contaminated yourself."

Then he skipped the second decon of the gloves. "Nope. Contaminated. You're dead."

Then he touched his wrist again. "Nope. You're dead."

Then his goggles. "You're dead."

Every time another mistake.

"You're dead."

Each time the same result.

"You're dead."

22

If there was a quiet intensity hanging over Cartersville that afternoon, the mood in Monrovia was simply intense. In fact, from Linda Mobula's point of view, all hell was breaking loose at ELWA. When she wasn't suited up and treating Kent at his house, she was suited up and treating patients in the Ebola treatment center. Every day, seemingly every minute, more cases were appearing in the city. The ETC was overrun when she had first arrived here, and it had only gotten worse since. The staff, stretched too thin already, was stretched thinner still when Dr. John Fankhauser came down with a fever and had to be quarantined. In Fankhauser's case it would eventually prove only to be exhaustion, but the mental toll was nearly too much for the staff to take.

This feeling was only amplified by the condition of their sick colleagues. Kent was in increasing amounts of pain. He was short of breath, often lethargic, and his telltale Ebola rash was getting worse. Where before

Linda had listened in on the long and wrenching phone calls between Kent and his family back home, now he was frequently too weak to talk for more than a few minutes. Linda was also caring for Nancy, who'd been diagnosed later but was older and whose illness had caught up with Kent's. Her symptoms were essentially the same. Linda didn't think either Kent or Nancy was about to crash, but nor could she say how long they would hold on. And so she wasn't surprised when she learned that Lance Plyler had started looking for an alternative treatment.

As disaster response team leader, Lance was sensitive to the well-being of his staff. Morale was already low. They might never recover from the shock of watching two of their own die. With all this in mind, Lance had concluded that rescue may not arrive in time and that saving their colleagues may fall to them. He began searching for something more potent than hope, which at the moment was all they had. He quickly stumbled upon something, and after a little cajoling it was now here, in his hands. The medication was drastic and more than a little dangerous but also, in light of everything going on around them, quite possibly their only choice.

The drug was called ZMapp. It was the product of a ten-year collaboration between laboratories run by the US and Canadian governments, along with a San Diego–based company called Mapp Biopharmaceutical, and together they'd come up with several different Ebola treatments. But it was ZMapp that showed the most promise. In early tests, the drug had a perfect track record and had cured Ebola 100 percent of the time…in monkeys. ZMapp had never been used in humans and in fact nobody knew what it would do inside the human body. There were significant and well-founded fears that it might trigger a deadly anaphylactic reaction. Under normal circumstances no one would even *consider* giving it to humans for years and then only after extensive drug trials. But then came the West Africa epidemic.

Seven courses of the drug—each course included three separate doses—had been set aside for emergency use if a medical provider were to get sick while treating patients. Those courses were shipped around the world to the organizations and governments fighting the outbreak. Course Two had originally been sent to the MSF camp in Sierra Leone, packed and sealed inside a white Styrofoam cooler. Through an extraordinary set of circumstances, it'd left the MSF camp, been flown through a monsoon in a small plane and canoed across a river and delivered to Monrovia—packed with dry ice and kept at –20 degrees Fahrenheit—and now, finally, was sitting like a time bomb in Lance Plyler's office.

The moment the drug arrived Lance felt tremendous pressure to use it, but also trepidation. Nobody knew what it would do to a person. Lance sought the advice of Lisa Hensley, a doctor from the National Institute of Allergy and Infectious Diseases. Together they called the head of Mapp Biopharmaceutical for information on ZMapp and then called an informational meeting with the ELWA providers. Linda did not attend. Though she was treating both Kent and Nancy and in theory the drug had been brought here to be used on one of them, she couldn't imagine a scenario where things got desperate enough to actually administer it. If little was known about Ebola in July 2014, even less was known about this drug.

When the cooler had first arrived, Linda found a paper published in a scientific journal that described ZMapp as a combination of mouse and human antibodies grown on tobacco plant bacteria. When given to infected animals, the antibodies had proven incredibly effective in fighting the Ebola virus. But the tests were in the very early stages and, again, conducted only on guinea pigs and monkeys. Linda had done medical research, had published papers, and knew the steps of bringing a new treatment to market. It's a long and thorough process of testing theories and correcting mistakes, of weighing risks against benefits, and this drug hadn't come anywhere near meeting that threshold. She didn't think, even in an emergency, even under compassionate care, that it would be used. They just didn't know enough. And so, since ELWA was literally overflowing with Ebola patients, Linda decided the best use of her time would be to skip the meeting and instead treat patients in the ETC.

She wasn't the only one having doubts.

Word of the drug had made its way to Kent and Nancy, who were sick and alone and scared. From her bed, Nancy picked up the phone and called Kent. Neither had much energy, and when he answered she got right to the point.

"Kent, are you going to take it?"

"I don't know."

"Well," Nancy said. "I'm gonna do what you do. If you're not taking it as a doctor, I'm not taking it either."

After hanging up, Kent lay in bed thinking. Whatever decision he made, he'd be making it not only for himself but for his coworker and friend as well. Time was inching on and they were both getting worse. He called Lance. Sick, scared, and isolated, his family halfway across the world, Dr. Kent Brantly told Lance he would be willing to take the ZMapp. He was volunteering himself to serve as guinea pig should the moment come, all the while holding out hope that, with an airplane on the way, it never would.

23

They practiced until they could go no more. Until they weren't thinking straight and were making mistakes out of pure exhaustion. In the run-up to other missions, later in the Ebola outbreak, Vance would sprinkle everyone's PPE with a fine powder and use a UV light to see where contaminate had gotten through, but for now all they could do was guess where the problems might be. The gear they would wear and the specific sequence in which it should be taken off were constantly found lacking and repeatedly modified. And still they didn't feel ready. They kept practicing. Then they practiced some more. Suits on, suits off, then back on again. They repeated the steps, all thirty of them, called them out, believed in them. Worried their way like monks around the rosary of donning and doffing. One problem they could not address was how the goggles and hood left exposed a portion of the forehead just over their eyes. They added a face shield but it felt flimsy—anything splashed or sprayed from the patient could get under it.

It was a problem with no fix. The product of an environment, equipment, and timeline that were all flawed. But you've got to accept at some point that you're taking a calculated risk and they had reached that point. And it was late, they were exhausted, it was time to call it. They left for the night but agreed to return if word came in about the flight. Jonathan went home and showered, then later drove his daughter Maddie to a cheer competition. The flight was weighing heavily on his mind and he looked through the windshield toward the sky and said to God, to the universe, to whoever was listening, *If I'm supposed to go, just send me a sign and I'll go*. It wasn't thirty seconds before his phone rang. It was Vance.

"Okay," he said. "We're wheels up tomorrow morning."

Jonathan hung up then looked back out at the sky. "Seriously man? I mean, you didn't have to answer *that* quick."

An hour away on the east side of Atlanta, Dr. Mike sat alone in his house. Worrying. He had faith in the protocols and in his people, in their ability to do the work they'd all done so many times before. But then,

Kent and Nancy had probably felt the same way and yet had gotten sick anyhow. He had no idea what had gone wrong at ELWA, where their system broke down, and whether the problem was avoidable or inevitable. He couldn't help but wonder if Kent and his colleagues had overlooked something simple but deadly and, if that was the case, maybe he'd done the same thing too.

24

Thursday, July 31, arrived gently in Cartersville. The sun rose at 6:30 but carried none of its usual menace. The high reached just 84 degrees, and on a day where precipitation historically averages nearly five inches, not a drop of rain fell. A light breeze blew out of the east but had no clouds to chase and instead drifted aimlessly across the open blue of the sky. Into this turbulent season of sudden rains and gusting winds, of mile-high thunderheads that spin moisture from the Gulf of Mexico into claustrophobic humidity—a torpid time, the time of tornadoes—there arrived a perfect summer day. Flying weather.

Pretty much what came to mind when Brian Edminster was asked to captain the first Ebola flight was *This is crazy*. And it was; it was crazy. Or it would've been, anywhere else. At Phoenix Air it was the kind of thing he almost expected. Edminster, age forty-two, had gotten the flight bug at six when his grandfather took him up in a corporate jet for the first time. The gauges and dials, lights, switches, the roar; he was hooked. He was green when he showed up at Phoenix in 1995, just out of flight school, and he learned how strange a place it could be when they sent him to attack the cornfield battleship.

Picture four jets. Late at night. Flying low over Manhattan on their way south to McGuire Air Force Base just east of Trenton, New Jersey. There's a fake ship at McGuire, in a cornfield, protected by the same radar systems that protect real ships. The military has a contract with Phoenix to test those systems. The pilots swoop in all night, changing the direction of attack and spitting bits of aluminum from the back of the aircraft to confuse the radar. There's no autopilot, just hand-flying for hours in tight formation. Bogeys over the Pine Barrens. It's dangerous and challenging flying, but at least no one's shooting at them. Phoenix also has a contract to help Navy gunners practice their marksmanship, and Edminster is one of the pilots assigned to drag targets out over the Pacific. On those flights he's primarily shot at with two different weapons. One is the CIWS (pronounced *see-whiz*), a ship-mounted gun that shoots 20mm shells at a rate of fifty rounds per second—it's not even a *bang* at that point but a *buzz*. He also drags targets for the Navy's five-inch guns, coming in 1,500 feet above the deck, low enough he can feel the concussion of the blasts coming up through the floorboards of the jet. Getting shot at in a small aircraft takes someone different, someone closer to outlaw than airline pilot, someone whose mindset extends beyond the practical considerations of mechanical flight and veers toward exhilaration. Edminster's got intense eyes and a deep voice and for years he'd been that guy.

As soon as he was asked to serve as captain of the Ebola flight, Edminster threw himself into flight planning. He studied the weather in Cartersville, out over the Atlantic, and also at his destination in Monrovia. He scanned a site called NOTAM, which gives up-to-the-minute information from airports all over the world. Weather delays, runway closures, the entire country falling prey to hemorrhagic fever—anything that might affect getting into or out of an airport can be found on NOTAM. He also called the FBO in Cartersville with a fuel order. Calculating how much fuel you can take on and still get off the ground requires factoring in several variables, including the aircraft's weight and local atmospheric conditions, plus runway length. This is not a casual exercise. Seconds before lifting into the air, a jet reaches V1—the speed at which it's no longer safe to abort a takeoff and the pilot is committed to going. What Edminster had to determine was that, if he had a mechanical issue after reaching V1 and couldn't safely stop, would the jet be able to get off the ground and circle back for an emergency landing or would it be too heavy and instead crash into the field at the end of the tarmac. Take on too little fuel and you flameout before reaching your destination; take on too much and you overshoot the runway.

After putting in his fuel order, Edminster picked up his paperwork—flight logs, manifests, insurance information, and a fuel wallet full of credit cards valid in various African nations—then headed to the aircraft, where his copilot was already hard at work.

Copilot Henry Hiteshew figured this would be one of those weird missions the moment Dent called him into his office. Hiteshew was at the store getting food to throw on the grill when the call came in. He drove to work, went to the second floor of the Silver Palace, and sat down across from Dent, who got right to the point.

"We're flying into Monrovia, to get an Ebola patient," Dent said. Then, "Actually, we're going twice."

Hiteshew grew up in Venezuela, the child of an American expat and a Chilean national. They lived in a remote mining area, where the Orinoco and Caroni Rivers meet, and everyone got around in small planes. His father flew and so did his father's friends. Hiteshew started out young, as a crop duster, and had moved up to small jets by the time Hugo Chávez nationalized the mining and oil industries. The government seized company assets and sold them off to foreign interests. When Phoenix bought the jet Hiteshew had been flying, they offered him a job and he took it. His first flight was from Bermuda to Memphis, which got a little dicey because he had no idea how to cross the Atlantic and had never used the Trimble GPS system installed in the aircraft, but he figured it out on the fly and now here he was, being asked to copilot an Ebola flight.

He looked at Dent and shrugged. "Okay, yeah. That sounds like fun."

"Good." Dent nodded toward his closed door. "Everything's already in motion but we're keeping this quiet. So don't tell anybody. Your wife, nobody."

When Hiteshew got to the hangar on Thursday, he began running through his preflight check of the aircraft. He started with a thorough investigation of the exterior, checking tires and nose gear, looking for leaking oil or hydraulic fluid, making sure the plane hadn't been damaged in any way or that a bird hadn't built its nest in one of the engines. Once inside the cockpit he checked the gauges. Electrical, batteries, hydraulics. Tested the alarms for overspeed and landing gear so if there was an emergency the proper alarm would sound and they'd know what was wrong. All-in, there are over eighty critical items to check-off on a Gulfstream III preflight inspection, but Hiteshew had flown thousands of trips and had decades of experience and was able to go through the whole thing quickly and efficiently, so by the time Edminster joined him everything was in order and they were ready to go. Edminster threw his bag on the plane, clapped Hiteshew on the back, and shook his head.

"This is crazy, right?"

Hiteshew nodded. Crazy.

Shortly before takeoff, the med crew joined them on the Gray Bird. Normally, the vibe is college road trip—a bunch of friends piling in, everybody buzzing with the unknown—but this time was different. Jonathan, Vance, and Doug settled into the back with plans to resume practicing the minute the jet reached cruising altitude and to keep at it the entire ten hours to Monrovia. Up front in the cockpit, everything was now ready for takeoff. Edminster disconnected the small portable motor that had been powering the aircraft during preflight and started the engines. Then he flipped the switch that reversed the airflow and pressurized the ABCS. He taxied to the runway, turned, got clearance from the tower, and accelerated. A few seconds later the Gulfstream III Gray Bird, tail number N173PA, lifted off. The first-ever international rescue mission to evacuate an Ebola patient roared off into the sky with a wink of taillights as it disappeared into the blue.

25

Forty miles away at his house in the northeast Atlanta neighborhood of Morningside, Dr. Mike Flueckiger scrolled through the contacts list on his cell phone. Because he was the medical director, because he'd be overseeing rather than directly participating in the two Ebola evacuation flights, he had a full and clear view of the storm system that on the ground felt like a disorienting tempest. An operation like this one had multiple phases, each with its own challenges and moving parts, with hundreds of tasks, all of which under normal situations would be handled individually and in sequence. But the way this one had come together, its especially urgent nature, the fear factor, the resistance, the still unanswered question of whether it could be safely done—everything had been scrambled. There'd been so much frantic activity over the last forty-eight hours that Dr. Mike was maybe the only person involved who remained removed enough to find and catch details that'd slipped through the cracks. And a big one had, though he was only just now coming to that realization.

Earlier that day, sitting in his house and staring at the clock, waiting for updates that he knew wouldn't come, he'd gone back through the particulars and the goals of the operation, the idea that they were attempting to bring Americans home, and right there it hit him. Kent and Nancy weren't going home. They had Ebola. Both would be delivered directly to a medical facility with a highly advanced team of doctors and nurses possessing the expertise, space, and equipment to handle highly infectious diseases. There weren't many facilities like that in the US, but the one chosen for this operation happened to be only a few miles from where he now stood. And yet, despite the fact that a destination had been selected and the clock was ticking, Dr. Mike had still not heard from its director.

He found the name he was looking for in his contacts and pressed Send.

Not far away, Dr. Bruce Ribner sat in his office. Since 2000, Ribner had been the head epidemiologist at Emory University Hospital, the sprawling medical complex whose campus ended at the front gate of the CDC. In 2001, a year after Ribner arrived, a risk assessment of the hospital's infection control apparatus revealed a startling oversight: They were a literal stone's throw from the CDC and its four-hundred-plus labs dedicated to the research of serious communicable diseases—not to mention the doctors deploying to outbreaks and then returning to Atlanta—and yet Emory, the obvious destination for anyone from the CDC who got sick, had neither the staff nor the facility to treat them. This coincided with a realization within the CDC itself that other than the vague notion of evacuation to an isolation unit in Ft. Detrick, Maryland, the CDC had no effective protocol for treating a staff member who got sick in one of their labs.

These twin revelations resulted in Emory signing a contract with the CDC to establish a Serious Communicable Diseases Unit on the ground floor of the hospital. The unit was primarily funded by the CDC but staffed and run by Emory, which named Ribner the medical director. Over the next thirteen years, the unit prepared for any number of deadly pathogens, but Ebola was never really on their radar. That changed in February 2014, when Ribner began monitoring the outbreak in West Africa. Over the months, he remained alert, but not overly so. Now it was July 31, the day after his birthday, and his phone was ringing with a call from Dr. Mike. The two men were friends and neighbors, and Ribner answered what he assumed was just a casual call, a happy birthday maybe. It escalated quickly.

"Bruce, did you hear that we're heading over to West Africa to pick up two Ebola patients?"

"No, I hadn't heard that—"

Dr. Mike laughed. "Guessed as much," he said. "Well, the State Department's asked us to go to Liberia to pick them up. I figured you oughta know because they're coming to your unit."

A pause over the phone. Then, "What?"

26

Twenty minutes after taking off from Cartersville, Brian Edminster peered up at the gauges on the top panel and realized they had a problem. As a jet climbs, the airflow coming in pressurizes the cabin and builds what's called differential. At cruise altitude the differential inside the aircraft settles at about eight or nine PSI. By now the differential should've been halfway there. But when Edminster checked the top panel, he noticed it hadn't gone up at all—the cabin wasn't getting the air it needed. If the jet doesn't get differential, it doesn't pressurize and the air inside the cabin will resemble the air outside, which is too thin to breathe. The lack of oxygen would make everyone lightheaded and slightly euphoric at first and then, eventually, they'd pass out. Edminster looked over at Henry Hiteshew, who'd keyed into the problem as well, and they decided to level off at about twenty-five thousand feet. They hoped if the aircraft remained relatively low that it would pressurize on its own. For several minutes they flew north over the Eastern Seaboard, eyes on the top panel. But it didn't go up. Their aircraft wasn't pressurizing.

While the aircraft was telling Edminster there was a problem that needed to be fixed immediately, experience told him not to rush. Take your time, whatever your next move is, make sure it's the right one, the safe one. Execute your plan. Be methodical. Be cool. This was a mindset he'd developed over time and through repetition. Cut your teeth flying small jets packed nose to tail with heavy explosives and you learn very quickly to be cool. He'd once flown a pair of warheads, stored in pressure-sensitive aluminum containers, to get serviced. During takeoff the pressure changed and one of the containers expanded. It let off an ear-splitting *BOOM* and for a fraction of a second Edminster thought *This is it*. But he was alive and a little giddy and he looked at his copilot and yelled, "What are we *doing*?!" They flew across the country laughing the whole way.

Edminster told Hiteshew to go back in the cabin and see if he could isolate the problem. Hiteshew followed the sound of rushing air to the rear of the aircraft where it had been modified to reverse the airflow. Rather than going through the outflow valve, air was leaking out through the seals around the modified door. He placed a garbage bag over the door and it was nearly sucked out. He went back to the cockpit and told Edminster and together the two of them spent about an hour troubleshooting the problem. Everything had to be right, had to be perfect. They couldn't take any chances, especially with this mission. But here they were, flying above Atlantic City and about to bank out over the ocean in an aircraft that wasn't pressurizing and couldn't climb higher than twenty-five thousand feet. Edminster radioed Cartersville.

27

Bad news was beginning to pile up. Half a mile from Kent's house on the ELWA compound, Nancy Writebol had taken a turn. Her diagnosis came on July 26, her birthday, and the home she shared with her husband David was quickly turned into an isolation unit. The world receded. Illness took control of Nancy's body, carried her out on the powerful current of physiological collapse, and then slowly began to drag her under. It was a nightmare come to life. The lone bright spot was David.

Nancy and David dated in high school, married in 1974, and remained—decades after most marriages passed their expiration date—wildly in love. Their faith created a sense of service and it was this desire to serve that had driven the couple into missionary work. They moved around often and had already lived and worked in Ecuador and Zambia before arriving the previous August in Monrovia. Their relationship of more than forty years was the one constant. And now this. David had no medical experience but immediately stepped in as caregiver. He needed Nancy, wasn't prepared to imagine life without her, and yet here he was, facing that very possibility. That afternoon, he wrote an email to friends back home bearing the news that Nancy's condition had worsened.

Not far away, in his office, Lance Plyler sat staring at the battered Styrofoam cooler. For a supposed miracle drug, ZMapp had so far caused him nothing but anxiety. How could he give it knowing it might cause harm, but then again how could he justify having it and not using it while so many were dying without hope? The drug was simultaneously, impossibly, both too risky to touch *and* too precious to waste; the agent that might make all the difference—for one person. Which was the other rub. He'd been warned when the ZMapp arrived not to split the doses, that for it to work a single patient would need to get each of the three shots. That person, he'd already decided, would be Kent—partly because nobody knew what the drug would do to a human and Kent had volunteered to serve as a test case. But there was another, more calculated methodology at work—the cold reality of triage says you focus resources not only on the most critical patients but on the patients most likely to benefit. Kent was twenty-seven, healthy, and stood a puncher's chance of survival. At fifty-nine, Nancy had more risk factors and was less likely to recover if she developed complications. It hadn't been an easy choice, but there it was. Or was it?

Just last night he'd been summoned to Kent's house where he stood outside the bedroom window listening to Kent explain how he had weighed the same factors but arrived at the opposite conclusion—Nancy should be the one to get the drug. Lance exchanged a glance with Linda, who was inside treating Kent with fluids and electrolytes. Kent pressed on, insisting this wasn't just an act of selflessness but a recognition of the reality—Nancy needed it more than he did. And besides, Kent said, he was feeling a little better. There's no way to quantify a feeling, but even if Kent had improved, it might not have been an altogether positive sign. Over the last few days both Linda and Lance had watched Kent grow less active, unable even to speak on the phone for more than a few minutes. His pain had increased, his breathing was becoming faster and shallower. The rash now covered his body from head to toe, a sign—along with the blood in his stool and vomit—that he was bleeding to death from the inside. Given these symptoms, Kent's sudden change might not be positive at all.

Lance had told Kent he'd think about it and now, Thursday morning, he was still wrestling with the decision as the Atlantic surf pounded the beach.

28

Jonathan Jackson knew something was wrong the minute he saw Hiteshew walk into the cabin. He watched calmly from his seat as the copilot tried and failed to fix a critical but recently modified piece of equipment in an aircraft cruising along at a couple hundred miles an hour. It was a remarkable display of calm under fire, but then again Jonathan's relationship to flying is unique by almost any standard. He applied to work as a flight nurse at Phoenix Air without ever having flown. Not once. The first time he set foot on an airplane was for a twenty-six-hour flight from Texas to Saudi Arabia in a Learjet with an ICU patient. From there the flying never stopped. He'd landed in nearly every continent and seen hundreds of countries before he flew on a commercial airliner. The first time he did—a long nonstop from Atlanta to Rome, crammed into a coach seat and sipping a tiny Coke—he looked around thinking, *This is some bullshit and I am not okay with this.* His strange introduction to flight gave him not only an appreciation of small aircraft but also of the rare skills possessed by the Phoenix pilots.

There were times they'd flown through turbulence so heavy he thought the jet would flip. There was that time the windshield shattered and also the night the landing gear failed and they had to bellyflop onto the runway. These were scary moments and he understood, even as they occurred, that this could be the way it ends, but he never felt an overwhelming sense of doom. Mainly that's because the vibe coming out of the cockpit was always calm, and so long as the pilots didn't panic—and they never did—then he figured there was no need for him to panic.

But that doesn't mean he never thought about the risks. Because he did. And now, as air whistled through the modified door at the rear of the Gray Bird, he couldn't shake the feeling that maybe this was a sign that they shouldn't be doing this particular mission.

After the aircraft had launched out of Cartersville, Dent went home. He didn't fly, he didn't provide medical care, and so there was nothing for him to do until the flight approached US airspace in about a day and a half. No sense worrying about what you can't control, or that's what he told himself. But he had flight tracker software at home and could keep tabs on their progress.

Before he ever got the chance, a call came in from dispatch. The airplane was coming back to Cartersville. Given how much was at stake, what you expect at this point is panic, is fury, is pointing the finger of blame at anyone involved, from the engineers who modified the airplane to the pilots flying it. But being in aviation means resigning yourself to the unpleasant fact that something is always breaking down. Dent was actually a little relieved it'd happened now—at least they weren't somewhere over the Atlantic. All he could do was trust his maintenance department to find and fix the problem before it became a disaster. They already had disasters. In fact, where the jet would land when it returned to the US with its first patient remained an unanswered question, which frankly was a little disturbing. There are only so many burdens one person can take on, and a mechanical issue on this flight, however worrying, was one more than he could bear.

"Okay," Dent said before hanging up. "Just keep me updated."

29

News of the mechanical issue was not met with such ease at Samaritan's Purse. When dispatchers at Phoenix told Ken Isaacs, VP of government relations, the jet had turned around, he yelled, "You can't bring the plane back!" They explained to him that no one wants to be stuck in an aircraft that won't pressurize while flying a critically ill patient across the ocean, that they were doing all they could to get the flight back up in the air but for now, until the problem was fixed, it was grounded. It was a sound decision, the only decision, but its impact across the ocean on Lance Plyler was massive.

Lance had spent an uneasy night and now a long day with nothing to accompany him but the difficult decision of whether or not to use an experimental medication on one of his colleagues. Now this. With prospects for a rescue suddenly uncertain, Lance's decision got that much easier. He climbed into his truck and drove over to Nancy's house. He parked, got out, and stood near her window. Even from outside he could see the situation was dire. Nancy had all the same symptoms as Kent—the respiratory trouble, the exhaustion, the pain, all of the signs that she too was hemorrhaging. But Nancy wasn't twenty-seven. He couldn't account for why Kent felt better, nor did he know if his sudden remission was real or just a precursor to the crash. But he felt certain that of the two, Kent was the only one who could hang on until whenever it was that the airplane got here.

He decided to give the ZMapp to Nancy. If he was wrong and she was too far gone to help, then he might be condemning Kent, but compassion overrode the doctrine of triage. He grabbed the cooler and handed it to the doctor overseeing Nancy's care, Deborah Eisenhut, with instructions to remove one of the frozen vials and thaw it beneath Nancy's arm. That simple act—no longer waiting and deliberating but taking action—eased his mind. Or at least it might have if there wasn't an urgent text message waiting for him when he got back to his truck. It was Linda saying to get to Kent's house immediately. Something was wrong.

30

The surprise phone call from Mike Flueckiger had left Dr. Bruce Ribner with mixed feelings. Within days, the first of two Ebola patients from West Africa would be coming to his unit for treatment. This was exactly the sort of emergency Emory's Serious Communicable Diseases Unit had been established to handle. His team wasn't just ready for the challenge, they welcomed it. But there was now a tremendous amount of work to do and very little time to get it done. When not in use, the unit existed in a sort of clinical hibernation, and it fell to Ribner as medical director to stir its various parts into a high-functioning whole. Dr. Mike estimated the first patient would arrive on Saturday, August 2. It was already Thursday afternoon and still no one else had contacted Ribner. Not a word from Washington or from the CDC, from *anybody*. He had no update on the timeline or the condition of the patients, didn't even have confirmation they were actually coming. He was on his own.

The first thing he did was notify the hospital CEO and the unit's chief nurse that two Ebola patients being evacuated from Liberia were on their way. His tone was understated and blunt but nonetheless his call lit fires all over the hospital. Ribner next began alerting and assembling the staff. When the unit was first conceived in 2001, Ribner and other top Emory officials had put a lot of thought into the type of person they'd want for such an exacting role. Though infectious disease units in other hospitals forced all their ICU staff to rotate through, Ribner couldn't see the wisdom in compelling someone to work in such a dangerous, high-stress environment where safety and survival required constant vigilance and painstaking attention to detail. Who'd even want to work alongside a scared or careless colleague that'd been pressed into service? His unit would be all volunteer. They canvassed three Atlanta hospitals—Emory University, Emory University Hospital Midtown, and Emory St. Joseph's Hospital—seeking applicants to staff a dynamic research and frontline communicable disease facility.

Responses flooded in. Before conducting interviews, Ribner first reached out to each applicant's manager and coworkers. He wanted to know if this was someone capable of following protocols to the letter, of doing everything right, every time. He needed people with stamina, an ability to function under stress, and a willingness to play a complementary role as part of a team. Just as important, he wanted to know how self-assured the person was and whether they had the confidence to operate outside of the normal confines of a hospital's leadership pyramid. Ribner needed people who could operate horizontally—on a peer-to-peer basis even with providers who outranked them.

After significantly winnowing down the pool of candidates, the interviews began. Those who made it through that process were run through the donning and doffing procedures to make sure they had the dexterity and the wherewithal to function in the suit. Candidates who made it through were welcomed into the unit. They started out with seven infectious disease doctors and thirty nurses. Ribner had in the years since kept the unit fit through regular training exercises, in the lab and out in the field, that included day-long classroom sessions followed by likely scenarios: a patient with SARS who arrived at Hartsfield-Jackson Atlanta International Airport; a CDC employee freshly back from Angola with symptoms of Marburg.

Much of the staff had been working and training together for nearly fourteen years and now, as Ribner put out the call for them to assemble, their dedication showed—everyone immediately agreed to come in including several who, even though previous activations turned out to be false alarms, cut short their vacations. As the unit quickly spun to life, there seemed to be only one thing missing. Experience. Since its inception, the unit had functioned as little more than an insurance policy. They had studied and trained and prepared for a moment like this, but after more than a decade of readiness, they had never faced a real event.

31

It was early Thursday evening when maintenance announced they'd fixed the modified outflow valve, reinstalled and tested the entire system, and had the Gray Bird ready for takeoff. The flight was back on. The first leg would take them 3,158 miles from Cartersville to the Azores for a scheduled fuel stop at Lajes Air Base, and from there they'd fly another 2,500 miles into Monrovia. Once in-country—and this part they hadn't even talked about, not really—they'd have to stay there, couldn't leave, no matter the condition of the patient. They'd be stuck. Because the FAA, because regulations. Because unbreakable rules that said they had to remain on the ground for a full twelve hours. For crew rest. Which was a joke, really, because who'd be able to rest after touching down in the middle of a deadly outbreak. But there it was.

And now here came the crew. Just a few hours after aborting their first attempt they were back on board and ready to go. It was Thursday, July 31, 9 p.m. local,

1 a.m. Friday in Liberia, when flight N173PA pointed its nose down the runway and began to gather speed. Seated in the back, Doug Olson felt an uncharacteristic rush of emotion. The excitement, the challenge, the danger of the missions, all of this attracted people to Phoenix. But what kept them around was compassion and the drive to do what's right. Doug knew very little about the people they were preparing to rescue other than that they had risked their safety to treat patients in a low-resource, high-risk environment, and now that the tables were turned, providing the same for them was simply the right thing to do. But it came with tremendous risk. There was the chance of an accidental exposure—the doffing process was full of question marks—but his greater concern was giving someone else Ebola. How would he feel if it was his mistake that got the pilots sick or his family, if he started an outbreak right here at home? And then what of the second patient, or any *other* patient that might someday need help. All those patients would be left behind.

Keeping this mission under wraps wasn't possible, it was too big, it was Ebola. But they hoped at least to keep the noise to a manageable volume until it was over. What none of them knew as the plane barreled down the runway was that news had already gotten out. For months now the staff at ELWA had been fighting a lonely and losing battle against a mysterious virus.

They needed help but the world had remained indifferent. Until now. The story of a doctor felled during a desperate struggle to hold the line against invaders sweeping over the fortress walls was ready-made for the evening news. It was bravery in the face of certain defeat, it was heroic, and Samaritan's Purse used it to bring attention to the larger story, which quickly came to include the rescue mission currently underway. Questions of Who and How and (soon enough) *Why* inevitably led reporters to this small town on the outskirts of Atlanta where it was rumored an outbound flight would soon be leaving for Monrovia.

In the final seconds before the jet reached V1, when its wheels were still on the ground, Doug caught sight of something through the window that made his stomach sink. He leaned forward to get a better look and sure enough there it was. A line of news trucks at the end of the runway. A half-dozen reporters. Camera lenses pointed directly at the airplane. Doug tapped Vance's leg and pointed out the window as the jet passed directly over the trucks.

"I think the word's out," he said. "Whole world's going to know what we're doing pretty soon."

32

When the text came, Linda was in an emergency meeting. The Ebola Treatment Center was full; a dire situation had veered toward disaster. They were discussing how long they could hold on and what they'd do once they no longer could, when she heard the ping and looked down at her phone. It was from Kent. But this one was more desperate than anything she'd seen yet.

Linda please come my temperature is up to 105 I'm really not doing well.

She calmly excused herself from the meeting and then, once outside, took off at a jog. At Kent's house she quickly donned her PPE and entered. It only took a second, really just a quick glance through her fogged-up goggles, to know. Linda by now had seen enough patients to recognize when one of them was dying. That evening, as she walked in, it was clear that she was losing Kent. The week had been a roller coaster but now Kent's mental status was waning and his pulse was far too fast. Same for his breathing. It'd only been a few hours since she'd seen him last and he'd insisted then he was feeling better. It was shocking to see how quickly he'd deteriorated. She went through the list of available treatments—all had been given and each had failed. Something else needed to be done or they were going to lose him. Tonight.

Getting into and out of PPE was such a long process that they often stationed a second provider just outside the window who could receive and relay messages. Linda went to the window and asked that Lance be sent over right away. When Lance arrived from Nancy's, he came to the same conclusion that Linda had. Something had changed. Kent's skin color was gone, his eyes were rolled back in his head, and he wasn't just breathing rapidly but struggling even for those quick, shallow breaths.

Lance looked at Linda. "I don't think he's going to make it."

A quick discussion of their options (they had no options) led to the vials of ZMapp Lance had just left on Nancy's porch. Linda was still skeptical of the drug. Her research brain simply couldn't trust a treatment whose N was something like nine patients—most of them monkeys. She didn't like the idea of using it but the alternative was even worse.

Looking at Lance, she said, "We can't just let him die."

If that was meant to be an answer it sure left a lot of questions. What would they do about Nancy? Could they justify not giving her the ZMapp when it wasn't clear she'd survive the night either? How had they even gotten to the point where two patients on parallel trajectories, moving at different speeds, arrived simultaneously at the point of near death? The answer, if there was one, came in the form of another question: What if they split the doses? They'd been warned against this, that it would leave too little medicine to help either patient and instead might kill them both. But then again, the medicine itself might do that. Nobody knew. It wasn't a decision to take lightly, nor was it something they could afford to deliberate. Faced with two bad options you take whichever is less bad, and splitting the ZMapp was about as less bad as it could get. They had a plan but Linda had questions, the biggest being, *Are we really doing this?*

33

Bruce Ribner flipped a wall switch. The overhead lights blinked, once, twice, and an instant later the Serious Communicable Diseases Unit came to life. For the next several weeks his universe would effectively shrink down to encompass little more than this room. The unit was intentionally small and secluded to keep it out of reach and self-contained. It was on the ground floor of Emory University Hospital, on a far corner with its own restricted entrance. The treatment area was 622 square feet, set up for three beds but with the capacity to hold up to eleven. It looked in many ways like a traditional ICU—heart monitors, IV pumps, ventilators, oxygen equipment, a cabinet of pharmaceuticals—except for a few specialized items such as light-activated sinks so staff would never have to touch the handles. There was an autoclave machine—a stainless-steel trap hissing pressurized, superheated steam—so they could sterilize their own equipment. The unit was also outfitted with a negative-airflow system, overkill for Ebola, but in keeping with hospital policy on highly infectious disease, Ribner switched it on. And it would remain humming in the background until the last patient was released.

With the unit alive and the staff assembled, Ribner ran everyone through a quick protocol refresher. PPE was to include a Tyvek suit, booties, hood with face shield, personal respirator, and two pairs of gloves. Shoes worn under the booties were to remain in the locker after shift and never leave. Period. Hand sanitizer was everywhere and should be regularly used to clean hands and gloves. Emory was cleaned and disinfected by a vast army of housekeeping staff, but by previous agreement they wouldn't be allowed to enter the unit. All spills were to be handled immediately and aggressively by the nearest providers. These protocols, along with all the others regarding patient care and waste disposal, needed to be followed by all staff all the time. Ribner reminded everyone that they needed to police themselves. Someone would be with each patient every single moment, without exception. It's stressful and labor-intensive—Ebola patients lose liters of fluid a day. They needed to be vigilant to avoid their own mistakes and catch those made by others. It was time to put their years of training to use.

Ribner felt prepared for whatever came through that door but knew that, technically, they weren't.

The unit was conceived as a fully staffed and equipped facility for the study and treatment of deadly pathogens. Which isn't cheap. A large part of what Ribner did each year was convince the CDC it was money well-spent—not easy on a good year, when budgets were fat, but 2014 was a bad year. That spring Ribner had walked into the budget meeting aware the entire program was on the chopping block. He had made his pitch and managed to convince the CDC that Emory's Serious Communicable Diseases Unit was worth the price. Mostly.

Hospitals are laced with a web of pneumatic tubes running through, around, and behind the walls where vials of patients' blood, urine, and tissue samples are shuttled to a central lab for processing. For all the obvious reasons, nobody wanted Ebola shuttling around the hospital. The unit had its own lab adjacent to the treatment area, a small, hooded workspace where fluids could be tested on-site. The CDC's budget folks had decided to keep the unit but stripped funding for the lab. The dedicated lab was expensive and the thinking was that if hadn't been used in thirteen years then probably it never would be. But the past is an unreliable predictor of the future and so here was Ribner, a little over twenty-four hours away from the arrival of America's first Ebola patient, and the lab where his staff would process blood work had been shut down.

As he scrambled to undo the mess and get his lab back online, he couldn't help but laugh. For over a decade the federal government had indulged him as a sort of nerdy Noah building an ark for a storm only he could see coming, and they'd chosen this year—when the storm clouds finally gathered—to decide there would be no flood.

34

Lance raced across the compound to retrieve the drugs for Kent. Linda was left alone with her conscience. Here was her patient, lying in bed, clinging to life, and she'd just agreed to a treatment that might kill him. Or she could decide not to give him the treatment at all and kill him that way. There are scenarios you study and train and prepare for so that in the heat of the moment preparation eclipses nerves; and then there are times like this when it's all a toss of the dice and any outcome but a perfect roll means someone's life. *Impossible* seemed too optimistic a word for this situation. Whatever she did was arguably wrong, an isolating reality, and yet what she didn't know was that she wasn't alone. Just a few days before, doctors not so far away from where she now stood had agonized over the exact same question. In fact, they'd agonized over the exact same vial of ZMapp.

The dose Linda was about to give Kent had been brought to West Africa by Gary Kobinger, a Canadian scientist involved in the development of ZMapp, who had volunteered with MSF earlier in the outbreak. Kobinger brought the drug along as a personal insurance policy and left it, when he returned home, at the MSF field hospital—the very hospital where Dr. Sheik Umar Khan, the virologist from Sierra Leone, was taken when he tested positive for Ebola. When he'd gotten sick someone proposed giving Khan the experimental treatment. The very suggestion was fraught with ethical and medical dilemmas. It had kicked off a massive crisis of conscience and a wrenching philosophical battle not only within the camp, but beyond it as well. MSF adheres to a philosophy called distributive justice, which says that everyone, regardless of status, is entitled to the same level of care. Since no one else in the camp was being offered the drug, how was it ethical to give it to Khan? There was also the possibility that the drug might kill him—itself a serious concern that no one took lightly—but here it had the extra wrinkle of distrust borne from generations of exploitation and colonialism, and many feared that if such a revered doctor, a national hero, an African, was killed by an experimental treatment administered by white foreigners, that it would incite more violence against MSF workers.

When word was passed that doctors at the MSF field hospital were leaning against giving him the drug, Khan's friends and colleagues around the world weighed in over a series of heated conference calls. Everyone was passionate, both sides had a point, no one was wrong. An entire medicolegal study could be written about this one case alone, but ultimately the doctors at the camp decided not to give him the drug. He died soon after.

Khan's diagnosis had come about a week before Kent's. His funeral, complete with pall bearers dressed in full hazmat suits, was happening right at that moment, 170 miles away. Linda Mobula wasn't fully aware of what had happened in Sierra Leone, but as the person who'd be pushing the drug, she faced the same ethical and medical questions as they had. She knew there would be people coming in after the fact to criticize any decision she made, and that chief among the criticisms would be that Kent, a white man, got the drug while Africans in the ETC were dying. Linda had done studies on race-based health disparities and knew the issue was real and affected quality of care—not to mention quality of life. She'd seen it with her own eyes while working in Baltimore and then again in Haiti, treating Black and underserved communities, experiences that left her with misgivings and second-guesses, with questions of fairness and justice, of injustice, from Tuskegee and beyond, a river of doubt churning with the flotsam of cultural baggage that for so long had clogged the flow of care.

But she knew too that she would never give the drug to an African. Not under these conditions. Trust was already deteriorating. If an African died in their clinic after receiving an experimental drug from Western doctors it could be catastrophic. The problem was so complex, so completely devoid of right answers, of good answers even, she could easily have drifted into indecision. But then from beyond the window came the slamming of a car door and a few seconds later, Lance's face at the window.

After leaving Linda, Lance had jumped in his truck and sped the half mile stretch to Nancy's house. Two of the three vials were still in the cooler, frozen solid and completely useless. He needed the thawed dose in Nancy's room. Kent was about to die but Nancy's condition, though not good—not even in the *neighborhood* of good—was better by comparison. And there were two more doses, either of which could be thawed and then given to her. Lance didn't put on PPE, didn't have time for PPE, just yelled for the vial through the window. Inside, Dr. Deborah Eisenhut grabbed the ZMapp from under Nancy's arm, sprayed it with bleach, and passed it through the window to Lance. He triple-bagged the vial, sprayed it again with bleach, and dropped it in a bucket. Then he put the bucket in the back of his truck, climbed up front, and sped back across the compound.

Linda saw headlights hit the side of the house. She went to the window and there was Lance, holding the ZMapp. Off in the darkness waves slammed onto the beach. Linda reached out and took the cold vial into her hand.

35

News of Kent and Nancy, their illness and hastily conceived rescue, their impending arrival in the US, of Ebola on American shores, first hit the CNN website and caught fire from there. The story got loud very quickly. But down on the first floor of Emory University Hospital, tucked away in their forgotten corner, Bruce Ribner and the staff of his Serious Communicable Diseases Unit seemed sufficiently insulated. Emory itself is hidden from the rest of Atlanta, in a quiet village shaded by century-old trees. By pecans, magnolias, poplars, and dogwoods, lazy canopies that stretch across wide residential streets, an in-town refuge. And the architecture of the houses: brick bungalows, mock Tudors, Spanish Revival, the occasional appearance of Prairie-style—a university president should live there, a novelist, the fanatically put-together daughter of some long-dead Coke bottler. Of all places, here, where every street filters toward the square that unfolds before the fountain that splashes onto the university steps, he should've been safe.

But where, before, Ribner had been Noah, now he was Eve—cast from this silent garden for the sin of taking action, for a willingness to stand up and do the right thing. Which of course is forbidden fruit in the run-up to a Presidential election. Ribner and his staff were putting themselves at risk to save Americans in peril—the most obvious, the most human, ironically enough the most *American* thing to do—but with the primaries just over the horizon it was treated as an act of radical politics. It was dangerous and reckless and absolutely should not be allowed. Pundits, columnists, seasoned politicians, and people only aspiring to the role weighed in on television, online, and in the papers. They came from everywhere, from nowhere, a furious Greek chorus:

> Ebola patient will be brought to the US in a few days
> Now I know for sure our leaders are incompetent
> KEEP THEM OUT OF HERE!

These were only the first shots in what would become a running gun battle of ugly commentary, but right away Ribner knew he and his staff had wandered into the crosshairs of a peculiar strain of the American body politic. Not only were Kent and Nancy labeled as enemies but so was anyone willing to help them. When Ribner alerted hospital leadership that the unit would be receiving Ebola patients, the PR team began working with their counterparts at the CDC to put out a coordinated, rational message. But this wouldn't be a time for rationality, and almost on cue local, national, and international media outlets began converging on this otherwise sleepy corner of Atlanta. Looking out his office window that Thursday night as the first of what ultimately would be dozens of media trucks began to arrive, Ribner surrendered to the reality that his team's first true activation wouldn't unfold in private or even under the sober observation of the medical community, but in the chaotic glare of a media shitstorm.

36

Terceira is a 150-square-mile spit of volcanic rock jutting from the North Atlantic, part of the Azores archipelago, home to fifty thousand people. On its northeast edge sits Lajes Field. The runway was built in the 1920s, expanded during World War II, and now serves as a waystation for aircraft flying east from the Americas. It's where the Phoenix Air Gray Bird stopped for fuel. Whatever you're flying (modified Gulfstream III or 747), whatever your destination (Scottsdale or Liberia), whatever your role (captain or passenger), there are certain universals to modern air travel, and one of them is that the instant wheels hit runway, you turn your phone on. As the jet slowed and made its way to the fuel shed, everyone powered on their phones, immediately setting off a riot of pings and vibrations and those *yoo-hoo* whistles people set as text notifications. Up in the cockpit, Hiteshew asked Edminster if he'd seen any media at the airport when they took off and Edminster said yeah, that he'd seen three or four trucks, which he thought was strange but hadn't given it much more thought than that.

"Why?"

Hiteshew showed him his phone. A chain of texts, mostly from his wife. He left without telling her where he was going or why, and while they were crossing the ocean she'd turned on CNN and saw footage of him taxiing down the runway. An anchor had speculated that the aircraft was going to pick up Ebola patients.

Hiteshew shrugged. "I don't think she liked that too much."

Then Hiteshew's phone started ringing. It wasn't his wife this time, but his daughter, who worked at CNN and whose coworkers knew what her father did and had told her, "We need that interview."

"Hey Dad, are you flying?"

Hiteshew played coy. "No, I'm just hanging tight."

"Are you gonna fly?"

"I don't know. Why?"

She sidestepped things as long as she could, just calling, no big deal, Hiteshew evading the whole time, until she finally came out and asked if that was him on the flight. And Hiteshew, still thinking maybe they could keep this all quiet said, "You know I can't talk about that."

In the back of the aircraft Jonathan was looking at an almost identical chain of texts. The first was from his wife. It was a link to the CNN video showing the Gray Bird's takeoff from Cartersville. He immediately called her. She picked up on the first ring.

"Can we talk about it now?"

"Well, shit," he said. "Yeah, I guess you can talk about it."

37

Kent had known all day he was going to die. For a couple hours now, Linda felt it too. Whatever her reservations about giving an experimental drug, and they were considerable, she was out of options. Linda was in her Tyvek suit, in two pairs of gloves, feet squeaking around in rubber boots, goggles fogged up with the heat, with sweat. She walked to the edge of Kent's bed, and through her mask she asked him for informed consent. She knew Kent knew about the drug, had been advised of its risks and possible rewards, that it might cure him or kill or who knew what, and even though in that moment he was too sick really to fully grasp what was going on—probably too sick to remember it anyway—she didn't feel right pushing it without first explaining what was happening.

Linda looked down at him. "I'm going to go ahead and give you ZMapp if you're okay with it. Okay?"

It was impossible to tell what was going through his mind. His eyes were bloodshot and rolled back, he was breathing heavily, gaunt from the virus, covered in sweat, but he agreed.

"Okay," he said. Raspy. "Let's do it."

Linda drew up the drug. She paused, she said a prayer. Then she injected the ZMapp into a 750ml bag of lactated Ringer's IV fluid. She spiked the bag with plastic IV tubing, and after purging air from the line, connected it to a port in Kent's arm. In a hospital setting—and absolutely none of this dispensing of unapproved drugs would ever happen in a hospital setting—she would have an IV pump that would dispense the drugs at a precisely calibrated drip rate so it wouldn't be given either too fast or too slow. A precise drip rate is often the difference between whether a drug works or not, whether it's harmful or not. It's everything, in other words, and Linda didn't have the ability to properly run one. Instead, she had to calculate the drip rate in her head, tabulations that competed for attention against panic, against doubt, against everything she'd ever learned about medical ethics.

She calculated what she thought was probably the correct drip rate then glanced at the clock over the head of Kent's bed and waited for the second hand to reach twelve. As the clock slowly ticked its way toward doom, Linda thought about how she'd probably lose her medical license if something went wrong but also about how this moment was so incredibly unique, so horrible, that if they were going to do anything at all they had to do it now. Whatever led her to this moment, she was about to step into the path of history by becoming the first doctor in the world to administer an Ebola-fighting drug into a human being. The second hand reached zero and using her thumb Linda slowly turned the wheel on the IV tubing to release the medicine. Gently though. Just one drip at a time so she could count them going in and match the rate against the second hand, which already was sweeping its way down the face of the clock. Had she started too slowly? Too fast? How many drips was that—fifteen? Was that last drop number fifteen? And what if it wasn't? Had she actually calculated right? Her head was swimming with horror and self-doubt and the anticipation of something going wrong.

Speaking of which.

Linda turned her attention from the slow drip of the IV fluid to the drug bag sitting on the table and drew up a vial of Decadron—a steroid used to counteract the symptoms of an allergic reaction. She wanted to have it just in case, though she had no way of knowing if whatever the drug was doing inside Kent's body right now could, if necessary, be reversed by a single dose of steroids. The first minute had come and gone, the first several minutes—where did they go? She couldn't say. She stood watching for ten minutes, fifteen minutes.

The medicine inched down the tube one drop at a time. She was consumed by the drops, her thoughts kept time to them. *I don't want him to die.* Drip. *I don't want him to die.* Drip. *I don't want him to die.* Drip.

Despite all the stress, the abject terror, Kent didn't react or change or even move for an eternity. He just laid there as the medicine went in—drip—and then, without warning, he started convulsing. Not a seizure but a bone-breaking shiver, a kind of full-body tremor that doctors sometimes call rigors. Linda had seen this in patients with fatal infections and she'd seen it in the end stages of Ebola. Maybe that's what was happening now. Or maybe the drug was killing Kent. Linda wasn't sure what was wrong so she wasn't sure how to fix it. Looking up from the bed, Kent said, "I don't know how you're going to breathe for me when I quit, because I can't keep this up."

Linda had been having the same thought.

38

Somewhere over the Atlantic. The Gulfstream III Gray Bird rocketed toward the northwest coast of Africa. Flying over the ocean at night is an exercise in sensory deprivation. Darkness above, darkness below, nothing but an artificial horizon on a dimly lit cockpit dash to say whether you're flying level or heading straight down into two miles of cold ocean water. In the back, Jonathan, Vance, and Doug ran through the process. One at a time they donned their PPE, went into the tent, pantomimed all the moves they'd have to make to reach equipment and monitors from a perch close but not too close to their patient. Then they exited and began the twenty-minute process of doffing, their legs trembling, their bodies exhausted—nobody had slept much over the last two days—trying, and often still failing, to get out without accidentally exposing themselves. It was almost time to do this for real and still they had problems.

39

Linda tried to calm Kent and so did Lance, from his spot at the window, though both of them in that moment were looking for reassurance themselves. The convulsions continued and then, over the course of that first hour, gradually began to ease. The infusion had started at 8 p.m. and by 9, Kent's fever had dropped from 105 degrees down to 100. Almost normal. Linda was cramped with tension and had only just started what would be a long night—within hours Kent's fever would spike again—but for the first time in a long time she had reason to hope that maybe one of her patients might get out of here alive.

40

The airport was dead. That's the first thing Brian Edminster noticed as he set the Gray Bird down at Roberts International in Monrovia. There was no chatter from the tower, no planes taxiing for takeoff nor any others lining up on the horizon for final approach. Just his solitary Gulfstream III and all around nothing but empty runway stretching in every direction. Edminster taxied to the customs ramp and powered down the engines. It was early morning but not that early and Roberts International was a ghost town. It was the apocalypse. Two men had been left behind as a half-hearted rearguard and they appeared now, an immigration agent and a fueler, both in makeshift masks and dishwashing gloves, big white rubber boots, pointing out to Edminster where he should leave the plane and then wandering off like they never expected anyone to arrive and didn't know what to do now that someone had.

Inside the cockpit, Henry Hiteshew was already

calculating how long until they could leave. Over the years he'd touched down on secluded runways that seemed peaceful right up until the moment he powered down the engines and it got quiet enough to hear the not-so-distant pop of small arms fire—spillover from whatever trouble their patient had stumbled into. The med guys would want to leave the aircraft, go wherever the action was, but Hiteshew would stop them, saying, "If you go and something happens, then I have to stay here and I don't want to stay." He had the same impulse now but this time he had no choice. It was Friday morning in Monrovia, not quite noon, and they were stuck here until 1 a.m.

Which wasn't the most comforting thought. Even Doug Olson, as experienced and steady as anyone on the crew, didn't particularly want to be in Liberia, not right now, not with Ebola around every corner. Treating patients was one thing but walking around a hot zone, sharing space with Ebola, knowing every surface you touch and person you meet could be the one that kills you, it was—well, it was something you had to put out of your mind. So instead, he started gathering the gear. He shouldered his duffel bag and the med kits, which couldn't be left inside a locked aircraft on a blistering hot runway, then climbed with everyone else into a white van idling near the terminal. The side door slid shut, the driver put the van in gear, and they pushed off from the curb and into Liberia. Some of the guys had been here before, others hadn't, but the first thing everyone noticed was how quiet the place had gotten. How eerie. Nobody on the street, no other cars. Jonathan's experience told him that roads in African cities should be crowded with cars, with drivers swerving into oncoming traffic to pass buses or motorcycles, narrowly, casually, avoiding head-on collisions. Horns honking. Foot traffic, bicycle traffic. Indecipherable pop music floating up from a damaged set of car stereo speakers.

Not today. Today the country was shut down and the radio in the van was tuned to a news station, broadcasting a sort of breathless, up-to-the-minute accounting of the virus and where it had spread. How many were affected. How many had died. The morgues were full, the government was digging mass graves, the virus had taken the capital and fanned out across the countryside—a nation subdivided into 136 administrative districts, and one by one they were all falling to Ebola. They rode in silence, listening to broadcasters describe a situation that felt less like a public health emergency than an outright invasion. Their hotel was forty-five minutes from the airport, much of it through country roads dotted with small houses and big termite mounds, with general stores, with places where there should be people, where there should be kids—there are *always* kids—but instead it was quiet, desolate, nearly an hour of driving with nothing but *War of the Worlds* radio sending horror over the airwaves, everybody afraid and the six of them wearing street clothes in a hot zone.

Kendeja Hotel. Seventy-eight tiki-style cabanas on thirteen acres of West African coastline. A pool, a bar, the pounding surf under a leaden sky. Walking into a new place meant first cleaning off the old one, and as they climbed from the van, they were told to walk single file through shallow tubs of disinfectant before entering the hotel. Inside they found just two employees—a registration clerk and a lone bartender (both scared)—and one other guest—a doctor for the US military. Otherwise, nothing. Otherwise, it was *The Shining*. Lonesome. Spooky. But also festive. Surreal is how it felt to Vance, sitting on the beach at a tiki bar waiting for zero hour on their Ebola flight. But not so surreal as to spoil anyone's appetite. If an army marches on its stomach, then Phoenix Air is like an army with tape worm—everything revolves around food. They grabbed a table outside and ordered pizzas. Lunch took some time in coming—the bartender was the only person in the kitchen—and when he set it down they measured with their eyes the distance between the tips of his fingers and the edge of their food, wondering just how safe it was to eat anything prepared, cooked, and served in a country ravaged by Ebola. But this was Phoenix and food is food so they ate it, though Vance personally couldn't tell much difference between the pizza and the box it came in.

They tried to relax but the question of what unexpected challenges this flight may hold hung in the air, so they just went through it all again from start to finish, who'd do what and in which order from the moment they laid hands on the patient—still *the patient*, still faceless, still uncertain which of the two they'd pick up first. Vance ran through protocols, double-checking the steps, choreographing first contact, Jonathan and Doug pitching the sort of hypotheticals and worst-case scenarios that would change everything, and then Vance revising, adjusting, just trying to meet the challenge. They circled the whole thing a couple times and finally called it—they were either ready or they weren't. It'd been a long few days and everybody wanted to go someplace quiet where they could be alone to sleep or at least relax and so, hours before the most important flight of their lives, each headed off to his own tiki hut.

Jonathan couldn't sleep. Just laid there having those alone-in-bed, sky-is-falling thoughts. *Are we gonna do this right? Should we be doing this at all?* Before they'd left, Dent had kept insisting they were making history, and each time he'd said it Jonathan would think, *A lot of people make history and not always for the right reason.* When this was all over, which side would history say they were on? He thought about the loading process, how if the patient couldn't walk they'd have to use the automatic loader in the cargo door, which was the worst way to do it because someone had to perch themselves on the edge of the platform as it went up, and he pictured himself there, riding with the patient, trying to balance and not fall off or lurch over onto the stretcher and expose himself before the mission had even got going. If he did expose himself, at any point, how would he tell Doug and Vance? There was just so much that could go wrong.

In the next tiki hut over, Edminster couldn't sleep, so he clicked on the TV and there was his jet, tail number N173PA, filmed from the rear as it lifted off. He couldn't believe it. Halfway across the world and he was watching himself take off.

"Henry!" He had Hiteshew on the phone. "Did you see us take off? We're on CNN!"

In the last hut was Doug. Staring at the ceiling and thinking about everything they'd already done to get ready and all that still lay ahead. As soon as he'd gotten to his hut and was alone, he'd reached out to the staff at ELWA. From them he'd learned about Kent, about how the last twenty-four hours had been hell, that he had nearly died before receiving an experimental drug. And now Doug was sitting in bed, sweating, not sleeping, wondering what drug had been administered to Kent, and if whatever boost it gave him would last long enough for him to survive the long flight home.

41

Linda paced her house. She needed to rest, even if it was just a nap, and she had laid down but couldn't sleep. Couldn't even close her eyes, not with all the nerves and the fear and the adrenaline still coursing through her body. So long as her mind was racing she might as well do something useful. She headed back to Kent's place, climbed into her PPE, and sat with him.

Whatever the drug had done, it was working. Where before he'd been restless and in distress, now he was quiet. They talked, had what passed here in the heart of the world's deadliest Ebola outbreak as a normal conversation. Kent asked where she'd gone to medical school, asked about her family. When Kent started to tell her that he had a wife and children, that they were back home in Texas, Linda said she knew—she knew everything, had been there for all of it and would never forget, even if Kent would never remember. Linda kept a skeptical eye on him but he was stable, calm even, and she had other patients. She slipped outside, climbed out of her PPE, and went to Nancy's house.

It was strange. Nancy was decades older than the average patient in the ETC and had once been the major concern and yet, though critical, she remained relatively stable. It was the younger Kent who'd spent a day wobbling on the absolute edge of death and who'd now be leaving first. This meant Nancy would have to wait an extra two days for evacuation and so she was allotted the rest of the ZMapp. She'd received her first dose shortly after midnight. Linda was on her way to administer the second course now. When she arrived, she climbed back into her PPE and walked inside. Linda found Nancy's husband David, like always, sitting next to her. David never left.

He remained at her side even after her diagnosis was changed from malaria to Ebola, opting simply to live within the quarantine. He was advised of the risk, which really wasn't even a risk but a near certainty—if he stayed, he too would get sick. But David wouldn't budge. They'd been married forty years and he'd rather die here than leave Nancy alone when she needed him. Linda found this amazing but also agonizing. She didn't want him to get sick—Nancy and David had children, grandchildren—nor did she want another patient. Together with Lance, she sat him down and tried to get through. She looked him in the eye, held his hand, and said, "David, please don't do this." He just smiled, like he was at peace almost, like he'd been traveling all these decades just to arrive at this spot, for this very purpose. So they'd taught him how to get into PPE and also how to doff, and there he sat. On the bed, next to his wife.

As Linda prepared the infusion, she was guarded but not nervous the way she'd been with Kent. She hung the bag and calculated the dose, then stood there with David, who was anxious, as it dripped in. She stayed a while to monitor Nancy's reaction, which wasn't nearly so dramatic as Kent's. Nothing alarming happened but then nothing spectacular happened either. Her condition remained critical and concerning. She was weak, profoundly dehydrated, and bleeding. She had the same bruising as the other patients, the same bloodshot eyes. And though they didn't have the equipment to confirm it, Linda suspected that a deadly loss of electrolytes—particularly potassium—was wreaking havoc on Nancy's organs and would soon lead to heart failure. This is what passed for a stable patient—someone drifting inevitably toward death but drifting slowly. Linda watched Nancy and David for a moment through her fogged safety glasses, then quietly slipped out.

42

They met in the hotel lobby at 6 p.m. It'd been a sleepless afternoon and now Edminster, Hiteshew, Doug, Vance, and Jonathan all piled into the van and drove out across the monsoon-wilted countryside to the urban wasteland of the airport. Kent was scheduled to arrive at 11 p.m., and between then and now all the preparation had to be done. They divvied up tasks as they rode, distributing effort and attention so that when the moment came and they stood for the first time over an Ebola patient there'd be no question of details slipping through the cracks. Everyone understood that for all the stakes of the operation, its scope and scale, its growing international attention, if failure came it would arrive on an overlooked detail.

Halfway to the airport, they passed a slow-moving convoy of military trucks. Nobody paid it much attention, not at first, but it stubbornly remained in the rearview, turning with them into the empty airport, snaking across the vacant runways, past the silent control tower, and all the way up to the Gray Bird. When they stopped, the convoy rumbled to a halt. Soldiers fanned out across the tarmac. Hiteshew watched, in the flickering glare of emergency lights, as a Toyota pickup with a tarp-covered bed slowly backed toward them. Sprawled across the bed in makeshift PPE was Kent, still enduring what for him had already been a long and tortuous night.

When confirmation of Phoenix's arrival had reached ELWA, furious preparations began for getting Kent out of his house and to the airport, located an hour away. Kent was given a clean pair of scrubs and a surgical mask, then stuffed into a thick yellow Tychem PPE suit with the hood cinched tight. Next came the gloves and a heavy pair of white rubber boots. Several doctors, including John Fankhauser, had also geared up and helped get Kent out of his house and into the truck. Their colleagues, held back at a safe distance by a rope, stood waiting outside to offer words of encouragement.

Kent was eased into the truck where he lay on a bed of foam cushions tossed in at the last moment. Fankhauser stood looking at his friend, already dangerously dehydrated and now practically melting inside a rubber suit. It would be a long ride, and miserable, but Fankhauser saw no reason it should also be lonely.

"We need somebody back there in case Kent has a

problem," he said. Then, careful not to tear his suit, Fankhauser climbed into the bed of the truck, settled in next to Kent, and took his hand.

Whatever misery Kent felt in his home at ELWA, it was much worse at the airport. They'd arrived far ahead of schedule and Phoenix wasn't ready, which meant Kent would have to remain in the bed of the truck, sweltering in his rubber suit. Fankhauser started calling for the Phoenix crew to get Kent out of the heat and into the plane as quickly as possible. He was weak and febrile and dehydrated. Hiteshew listened to the exchange. He wasn't sure of the outside temp but figured it was over 100 degrees, easy, and Kent was lying there in full PPE. It must've been torture.

But nobody from Phoenix was dressed out yet and they still had to prep the jet and the ABCS. Whatever hope they harbored for an orderly procession of preflight work was gone and the race was on. In a sense, this was exactly why they'd spent the last few days planning and practicing, and also why they'd gone through it all again that afternoon over another cardboard pizza—to have everything agreed upon and committed to memory so when the moment arrived no one would have to think about their job, they'd just do it. Edminster was in charge of flight planning, and since no one from customs or air traffic control had shown themselves, he trotted off in the direction of the tower to get the jet cleared for takeoff. Hiteshew busied himself with the preflight checkoff. He completed his walk-around, then hopped in the cockpit to run through the checklist and fire up the auxiliary power unit. Until they turned on the engines, the APU would power the plane, cool the cabin, and pressurize the ABCS through the reversed airflow valves. If everything was working as it should be, a green indicator light would illuminate overhead. He flipped on the APU—moment of truth—and looked up. *Blink.* The green indicator light came on. ABCS was a go. Hiteshew climbed out of the cockpit and ran off to find the fuel tech.

In back, the med team was scrambling to turn the jet into a biocontainment unit. They dragged in all of the gear they'd removed upon arrival, flipped on monitors, and connected lines and then, while the ABCS pressurized, turned their attention to the cabin itself. When Vance made his Tuesday afternoon Home Depot gear run, he'd grabbed plastic sheeting in varying thicknesses to drape the cabin so the interior wouldn't be contaminated. Through trial and error, they decided that nine-by-twelve sections of 2mm plastic sheeting worked best. Anything thinner was too flimsy, anything thicker too stiff. All-in it took two drapes per side, four total, running from the headliner, down over the seats and to the floor, where they overlapped and bunched underfoot. In the back of the cabin, the drapes hung from an overhead rail but up front, in the area around the door where the patient would actually enter the aircraft, there was nothing to clip them to. Vance rummaged through his bag, pulled out a fresh roll of duct tape and, with Jonathan's help, taped the sheeting to the cabin wall. By now the AC was pumping and the cabin had begun to cool, which provided relief from the heat but would shortly, though they didn't yet know it, start to work against them.

Outside, Hiteshew had tracked down a fueler but ran into another problem when the guy wouldn't pump their gas. Refused. Wouldn't go near the aircraft. He'd been told to expect only a plane, there'd been nothing said about a patient, about Ebola, but now there was Kent, stretched out in the back of a pickup, and the fueler wanted no part of this at all. Hiteshew told him it was safe. That the plane itself didn't have Ebola. He even offered to help pump, but every time the fueler looked at the convoy of trucks surrounding the pickup he'd step back a little farther, shaking his head and saying no, that he wasn't going anywhere near *anybody*, definitely not sick-looking people in PPE.

Hiteshew explained this wasn't negotiable, they needed gas. He stopped asking and flat-out begged the guy, but all he got in return was that shaking head, the feet slowly shuffling backward. Screw it. If the fueler wasn't going to do his job, he'd do it for him. Hiteshew ran over to the fuel truck, climbed in, and fired up the engine. He threw it in reverse and backed up to the plane, then hopped out and chocked the wheels. He grabbed the fuel hose, ran out enough length to reach the aircraft, and connected the line. Everything was set except for the fact that he didn't know how to pump the gas.

Inside the airport, Edminster had finally found somebody to run his flight plan through the system. Which for a second was a relief, but then the guy sat down at the computer terminal and with one finger started searching for keys. Slow-typer doesn't begin to cover it. The guy poked at the keyboard like he was checking to see if it was dead. Time stretched and expanded; it was the *minute* hand he heard ticking. They had to go, they *really* had to go. But there was no speeding this up. Each time Edminster looked down at his watch, the man would stop typing and glance up from the keyboard.

"I don't like to be pressured."

"Come on," Edminster said, "we need to hurry. This guy's sitting in the back of a pickup."

It was just the two of them in a room of blinking computer screens. Edminster stared. The man stared.

Then he returned to his keyboard. *Enter aircraft number*: N . . . 1 . . . 7 . . .

Down on the tarmac, Hiteshew turned to the fueler and held his arms up—without help they'd all be stuck here. Together. The fueler called out instructions and Hiteshew caught most of what he said but it was hard to hear over the noise of the aircraft and the fuel truck, and mostly he just kept an eye on the gauges hoping he didn't overfill the tank and spew jet fuel all over everyone.

Inside the jet, everything was finally ready for Kent, so the med crew climbed into their PPE. The world was an oven; they instantly started sweating. They lined up near the door to the aircraft, were about to step outside, when the draping around the door sagged, swayed, and fell to the ground in a giant heap. Vance stood there looking down at the yards of plastic sheeting piled up around his feet. It was the AC. The ambient air was so hot and humid that once the AC kicked in, the walls started to sweat and the condensation peeled the tape loose. So now they had to start all over again. Doug, Vance, and Jonathan, fully covered in Tyvek and non-latex rubber, scrambled to get it all back up. It took a lot of tape. An ungodly amount of tape. But it was up and with any luck it might hold.

Finally, they stepped outside. Vance was the first one

down, crinkling and a little unsteady inside his plastic cocoon. Mind racing. Tuesday was a lifetime ago, way longer than three frantic days, but the moment had arrived and he was nervous as he stepped out onto the tarmac. Fankhauser met them a few feet from the pickup and delivered a quick medical report. Jonathan stood off to the side. His eyes shot from Fankhauser to the pickup to the convoy of soldiers. He noticed they were armed. Jonathan had rescued injured Americans from violent places, countries in the grips of gang war, civil war, all-out war, cities where the ground rumbled with the distant *crump* of artillery, and even then nobody had a weapon. But here they were, nothing more dangerous than a virus, and fifteen people with AK-47s had been sent to make sure the patient got onto the aircraft. It spoke of the fear and hysteria in Liberia, and that made Jonathan think about the fear back home, about his wife and his daughters and how the world was finding out their dad was here, doing this.

As Fankhauser finished his report, Vance approached the truck. Kent was laid out in the back and not moving much. Even through the PPE Vance could tell just how weak and sick he'd become. His condition was serious but it wasn't something from a movie, it wasn't blood shooting from the eyes and liquifying organs and exploding torsos. It wasn't biblical. It was medicine. Kent was a patient and Vance was his nurse. In that moment the mystery lifted and he climbed into the back of the pickup and crawled forward until he was crouched by Kent's side. He took his hand.

"I'm Vance. We're going to take you home."

43

Dr. Mike needed to get out. There were only so many hours he could spend at home watching the clock or willing the satellite phone to ring (it never rang) with an update from the crew. He'd worked an emergency room shift the day before, which kept him occupied and made the waiting easier but here at home there was no escape, nothing to do except wonder where they were and how it was going. It was a strange position for him and brand new, to be the medical director but not on the flight—in charge but not *in charge*—totally vested but entirely unable to help. It was enough to drive him crazy. He tossed his mountain bike and some gear in the car. The woods, trails, speed, that's what he needed—put this whole thing out of his mind for a while, lose the anxiety to exhaustion. But it wasn't to be. He hadn't even made it out of the neighborhood when his phone rang. Dent was on the line and fired up.

"How fast can you get up here?"

For the past week Dent had been so busy getting this mission off the ground that he hadn't stopped to consider how the general public might react to it. The answer to that, it turns out, was not well at all. The minute news broke that Phoenix Air was about to bring home the American doctor who'd contracted Ebola—a man whose slow, agonizing death audiences had been following on television—the whole world turned upside down. The half-dozen cameras camped at the end of the runway when the Gray Bird took off for Monrovia were only just the beginning.

Before Vance ever crawled into the back of the pickup truck to begin treating Kent Brantly, Phoenix Air was under siege. The phones started ringing and never stopped. News trucks surrounded the building and clogged the road running between the Silver Palace on the west side and the airfield on the east side. Live feeds were broadcast from the edge of the parking lot. There were so many cable news reporters crammed into Moore's Gourmet Market on Fite Street in downtown Cartersville that come lunchtime you couldn't *buy* a table. With the added attention came added scrutiny, and now everyone was questioning not only the wisdom of bringing Ebola patients back to the US but also Phoenix's ability to safely do so. It wasn't long before the grumbling reached Dent's payroll.

Phoenix employees pride themselves on an ability

to pull off the dangerous and the impossible. It's part of why they work there. But they're also human and, along with their spouses, they'd been watching the news and heard the pundits. A flicker of doubt within the walls of Phoenix Air grew into a flame that by Friday fueled the burning question of whether all this was actually a good idea. To head off a mutiny, Dent called an emergency meeting for any employee and their spouse with questions, concerns, or flat-out refusals—*whatever you got, come on in and speak your mind.* He planned to run it but he knew the only person anyone really wanted to hear from was Dr. Mike. Speaking to him now over the phone Dent was anxious.

"I need you to get up here."

44

Henry Hiteshew was witnessing a miracle. Their patient, a young doctor whose name he just learned was Kent Brantly, slowly rose from the bed of the makeshift ambulance and stood on wobbly legs. There were two ways onto the Gray Bird, and rather than be lifted through the cargo door Kent insisted he could walk up the steps. Vance and Doug lifted and eased him down onto the tarmac. Vance was in front, Doug behind, both holding and steadying Kent as he extended one rubber boot in front of the other and began to walk. His gait was stiff and uneasy, like after a week in bed he'd forgotten the choreography of motion. Hiteshew watched through a rising curtain of jet fuel vapors as the apparition—two men in gleaming white Tyvek, a third, skeletal in dingy rubber—approached his aircraft.

Hiteshew didn't know much about the virus but he was certain as he watched them carefully guide Kent into the plane that both Vance and Doug were in incredible danger. Especially Vance, who Kent clung to as he trudged up the steps and onto the aircraft. The Tyvek could tear or a sleeve could bunch up, Kent could suddenly and without warning vomit a stream of infected blood directly onto Vance, and then what. Hiteshew's heart was pounding as they walked over the plastic draping and eased their way into the ABCS. Outside, a pair of men in white suits sprayed a bleach solution over the path they'd just taken from the truck to the aircraft. Hiteshew watched as Kent was settled into the ABCS. Kent was pouring sweat and looked exhausted, but his eyes were what drew Hiteshew's attention—they were bloodshot and unfocused, fixed on a spot in the middle distance. It was a look he'd seen before, ominous, what he called the death stare.

45

A maintenance hangar was cleared for the meeting and outfitted with chairs, a stage, and a microphone. About a hundred and fifty people showed up and by the time Dr. Mike got there the place was buzzing with a nervous energy. Neither he nor Dent had prepared anything; the plan was to be as candid and honest as possible, just to lay it all out and then listen to whatever everyone had to say. The two of them walked in together, and as they took the stage the crowd fell into an anxious silence. Dent spoke first. He talked about the Friday phone call from Walters, the Tuesday meeting with the government scientists, and the situation in Liberia. He talked about the ABCS and the work that went into creating it, about its remarkable capabilities, and how really the system was overkill for what they were facing. Dr. Mike was next. He talked about the training they'd done and the protocols they created, all the safety measures in place to protect the medical crews, the pilots, maintenance, everybody. He explained how the virus was transmitted, tried to debunk some of the myths surrounding it, but even as he talked, he could feel pushback, a restlessness hanging in the air. Like all this was fine, but not really what anyone had come to hear. He felt Dent had sugarcoated it a little and now here he was being technical, and he understood instinctively that neither approach addressed head-on the central issue, which was fear.

"What questions do you have?"

A voice from the middle of the hangar: "Can we do this safely?"

Dr. Mike wanted to be as honest as possible. Many of the people seated in the hangar had come to him over the years for medical advice; they trusted him. As if that wasn't pressure enough, he felt the added weight of knowing that if it turned out he was wrong in approving this mission, his mistake might make any one of them sick. On the question of whether or not they could do this safely, he gave them total candor.

"I don't know for sure if we can," he said. "I believe we can, otherwise I wouldn't have signed off on it. I believe in it enough that I'll be getting on a flight."

Someone asked how long the virus could survive on contaminated aircraft components and if by working on them they should be concerned about getting sick themselves or, worse, bringing something home to their families.

Dr. Mike looked out over the hangar, at all the faces staring up at him. "I'm scared," he said. "For my own safety, for your safety. But it's only going to make us that much more careful. My family is just as anxious as yours. My daughter's a bit of a hypochondriac. She'd prefer I wasn't doing this, but it's what we've been training for."

This drew pushback from several people, who said this wasn't what the tent was designed for. He held firm: "This is exactly what it was designed for. We're going to do everything possible to keep it safe and if that ever changes, we'll stop."

"But why do this at all? We've got so much other business."

He nodded. "That's true. But it'd be very difficult to have this asset and say 'no, we're not gonna use it.' "

Dr. Mike felt that about half the crowd was with him. Maybe 75 percent. Which, honestly, felt about right to him. This mission carried very clear risks and required courage from everyone involved. Few of the people sitting before him had any medical experience and even fewer understood Ebola. They were right to be scared, the world around them was panicking, but instead of walking out they'd come here to listen. It was bravery in the face of uncertainty, which Dr. Mike felt spoke to Phoenix's sense of service. And he appealed to that now.

"We're not being forced to do this," he said. "But in the largest sense of the word, we're *obligated* to do it." Then, in that soft voice you have to lean forward to hear he said, "Because we have the capability to do it. And we should do it. It's the human thing to do."

46

Sealed inside the ABCS, isolated by multiplying layers of PPE, buffeted by air whistling through the filters, Vance was an astronaut on a moonwalk. After stripping Kent of his PPE, he put him in a lightweight set of paper pajamas, then shuffle-stepped him toward the bed. Standard nurse care really, except here if Kent fell or got disoriented, if he frantically reached out and tore Vance's suit, it could mean infection, and eventually death. Once he had Kent safely in bed, Vance connected a series of monitors that would track his blood pressure and blood oxygen levels, as well as his heart's rate and rhythm. He wanted to move slowly and with careful intention to avoid an exposure, but the clock was ticking. How long had it been—forty minutes, fifty? It felt like an hour. Not even done yet and already fatigue was setting in. The final step before takeoff was to start an IV for fluids and meds.

Piercing a vein with a needle is difficult on any patient. Veins can be hard to see and sometimes even if you can see them they're small and spidery and burst the instant they're stuck. Sometimes they roll away from the needle. There are peculiarities in anatomy, pliancy of the flesh, an individual patient's reaction to a needle coming at them, and the steadiness and competence of the provider themselves. All this and more on a healthy patient, but Kent wasn't healthy. He was beyond dehydrated and had started third-spacing, a phase of illness where the fluid leaches from the circulatory system to pool in the soft tissue. Vance wrapped a tourniquet around Kent's forearm, swabbed the inside of his elbow with an alcohol prep, and grabbed a needle. He'd started a thousand IVs in his career, a million, hardly even thought about it, but this one was different.

With two pairs of gloves, he had no dexterity. It would be so easy to stick himself with the needle but no, he couldn't even think about that. He focused instead on the task, how Kent needed this IV for fluids and pain meds and anything else Doug wanted to hang during the flight, and then there was the possibility that Kent might go into heart failure or respiratory failure, even full cardiac arrest somewhere out over the Atlantic and then he'd need a whole pharmacy's worth of drugs. All of them given by IV. They needed this line.

Vance caught sight of a vein on Kent's arm. He

had the needle over the site, hovering, but now the moment was catching up with him. The stakes but also the heat. His mask was fogged up and he was nervous. Bent at the waist, legs trembling. He blinked away the sweat and in went the needle. A flash of blood in the chamber let him know he was in, and he advanced the catheter into the vein. He tossed the needle in their sharps container and connected the IV bag.

Up front, Hiteshew was anxious to go. Brian Edminster had finally gotten their flight plan entered and approved and was back now, sitting at the controls in the left seat of the cockpit. Hiteshew glanced back at the ABCS and saw Jonathan Jackson guiding Vance through the doffing checklist. They were as ready as they were going to get. Time to go. Hiteshew jumped out, disconnected the fuel nozzle, retracted the hose, and then backed the truck away from the plane. He ran around the jet, kicking away the wheel chocks and making sure they were clear, no cones around the engines, nothing near the wings. He motioned for Edminster to fire up the first engine, then jumped back in the airplane. Edminster started the second engine and they were taxiing toward the runway now, no other planes in sight, air traffic control coming in over the radio to say they were clear to go and keep on going, don't come back, not with that cargo. Everyone in back was seated and buckled. Edminster had them pointed down the runway, throttle down, picking up speed, Monrovia turning to a blur outside their window, and then he pulled back on the yoke, front wheel off the ground, and they were up. Aircraft N173PA was in the air and on its way back to the US.

47

Dent returned from the emergency meeting with his employees in the maintenance hangar only to learn that while he had been off putting out that fire another had sprung up in its place—no airport on the East Coast would allow his jet to land. The record scratched. The world froze. Even Dent—a fountainhead of conversation, opinion, and anecdotes delivered with the effortless, perpetual sweep of Swiss time—fell silent. Twenty-four hours prior, as his crew departed Cartersville for Monrovia, Dent had secured tentative clearances for their return. He had spoken with officials from the airport authority at Bangor International in Maine and also their counterparts at three airports in Atlanta—Peachtree-Dekalb, Hartsfield-Jackson, and Fulton County. Agreements had been reached for the aircraft to land at Bangor for US Customs, refuel, and crew swap, before heading south to Peachtree-Dekalb where a ground crew would transport the patient to Emory. Simple. Easy. Nothing they hadn't done countless times before and once with a nuclear bomb. But a jitteriness had set in among his partners. Here, in the eleventh hour, was the specter of failure that had haunted his sleep since that first call from Walters.

Ebola was no more deadly than a handful of other horrible viruses that occasionally emerge from nowhere but, like yelling *Shark!* at the beach, the very word inspired an outsized and paralyzing fear. Until now it'd been an ocean away, but the mission to bring Kent home changed that. Suddenly Ebola wasn't just *there*, it was *here*, this horrible, deadly disease—have you seen *Outbreak*?!—was on its way. All that we didn't know or misunderstood about the virus metastasized into fear, and fear is the easiest emotion of all to harness. Kent was no longer just a doctor or humanitarian, an American, he was a threat, the carrier of a deadly and mercurial virus. The second he set foot in the US he'd become patient zero, and how was *that* a good idea? Again the Greek chorus of influential voices took to social media:

> The U.S. cannot allow EBOLA infected people back.
> People that go to faraway places to help out are great—but must suffer the consequences!

That two of their fellow citizens should just be

left overseas to die was a remarkable stance for any American to take and the opposite of what the US practices every day. When the thirty-two-foot sailing vessel *Satori* sank in a mid-Atlantic gale in the fall of 1991—an event Sebastian Junger immortalized in his book *The Perfect Storm*—rescue efforts included jets from both the Air Force and the Navy, multiple helicopters, a Coast Guard cutter, a team of rescue divers, and pledges of cooperation from every shipping vessel within radio range. All this to bring home three Americans who'd run into trouble while undertaking nothing more important than a pleasure cruise. And yet a doctor trying to stem the tide of a deadly virus should be left to die where he fell.

It's an unfortunate footnote to human history that we're motivated more by fear than reward, but the evidence was there to see as the voices multiplied and got louder:

> Can't anyone serve Christ in America anymore?
> Ebola doc's condition downgraded to 'idiotic.'

Aside from the fact that pundits were blaming Kent and Nancy for their condition, speculation arose that terrorists might get ahold of Kent's urine and use it to expand the already frightful world of biological weapons. Hysteria had officially arrived.

And it was every bit as contagious as the virus itself. When Dent got to his office, he found messages from all the Atlanta-area airports saying they'd changed their minds and that no jet carrying Ebola patients would be given clearance to land. He got the same call from the airport authority at Bangor International. After that, Dent's phone never touched the cradle. He rang up other airports in other cities and at the same time was putting in calls to Walters saying that every possible avenue for a landing site on the East Coast was shutting down. His crew had already taken off; the flight was underway. The aircraft would be here in twelve hours and it suddenly had no place to land.

48

Doug Olson stood as the Gray Bird reached cruising altitude and began suiting up for his first shift in the ABCS. Once inside he performed a quick assessment on Kent. The humidity in the aircraft was extremely low and, after so much time in the tropics, was a shock to Kent's severely dehydrated body. He was completely dried out. Doug checked vitals, hung more fluid, pushed electrolytes and nausea meds, and offered something for pain. Kent was comfortable but weak and mostly slept. Doug, Vance, and Jonathan rotated in and out. Doug would ultimately take three turns inside the tent, but this was his first and he didn't yet know his limits. He was used to hands-on care and wanted to constantly monitor his patient—something the ABCS prevented—so he remained inside for an hour. Which was too long. It wasn't the work that was difficult but the conditions. It was incredibly hot inside the PPE and Doug was sweating profusely and hadn't slept in days. The whole time he was in there his body was getting weaker, exhaustion slowly creeping up, and when it all finally caught him, it hit with the force of a hammer. Energy and focus were leaking from every pore. He needed to get out before he made a mistake. He turned toward the door.

All he wanted was to sit down but his gear was contaminated and dangerous and would need to be removed through their painstaking doffing process. Already he was almost too tired to try. They'd discussed this in practice. But it's not until you're in the tent with a real patient, no easy way out, that you fully appreciate just how taxing it is. The key was to leave early while you still have energy. It was too late for that now. By the time Doug reached the antechamber he was pouring sweat, hyperventilating, and slightly light-headed. His legs were shaky and unsteady. He'd arrived at the most dangerous part of the mission both physically and mentally drained. He was used to dangerous. He'd done it, in Yemen, where he deployed in the fall of 2000 as part of an FBI task force investigating the bombing of the USS *Cole*. The country wasn't safe but he spent weeks there, much of it beneath billboards for the bin Laden family's construction company scouring sites where the bombers had planned and prepped the attack, at the spot where they stopped in a boat full of explosives to pray before detonating their bomb. It'd been an anxious, twitchy season, but this—bristling with Ebola and almost too tired to care—this was flat-out scary.

Outside the tent Vance began running through the checklist. Doug felt a concern for his own safety, for the safety of Vance and Jonathan, but also for the mission itself. He wanted not just to do this, but to do it right. A mistake here could cause an outbreak at home and that thought alone was almost enough to derail his concentration. Plus, there was the nagging voice of doubt whispering that this had never been done and that maybe the reason was it *shouldn't* be done. And though he understood infectious diseases, he wasn't an expert. Ebola was complicated, the transport and treatment process was complicated. Was there something they overlooked? It was all coming from so many different angles, from every direction, he could almost feel himself spinning out and—

"First inspect your PPE for cuts or tears."

Vance, outside the tent, began calling out the steps. Doug turned. He was tired and struggling and needed help—and now, there was Vance. All he had to do was follow the sound of his voice.

"Inspect your PPE for cuts or tears..."

Doug nodded, then began following the steps. Outside the tent, Vance continued calling out the steps—*Disinfect your outer gloves*—and leading Doug through the process that would ultimately deliver him back to safety. They both were tense. Before takeoff, Vance had come out of the tent in a live situation, but this was the first time anyone had ever done it while airborne. What if the jet rocked or dropped and caused Doug to lose his balance and brush an exposed arm against the side of the tent? His legs were already shaky, how much turbulence could he take before he fell? Just how steady could Edminster keep this thing?

However damn steady you want, is how Edminster would've answered that question. A few years before, a flight crew from the Alaska state patrol conducting helicopter surveillance of Cook Inlet spotted a seven-foot beluga whale beached on the shore. Help was called and the animal was brought to a local aquarium while a permanent home was found. That home, it turned out, would be in San Antonio, about four thousand miles away. Phoenix Air was contracted for the job and Edminster was assigned to the flight. He had piloted the very same Gulfstream III Gray Bird, with its rare and all-purpose cargo door, that he was flying right now. The whale was placed in an open-topped tank fitted with a sprinkler system. There was two feet of standing water in the bottom of the tank, and Edminster had to fly the jet nearly the entire length of the North American continent without any water sloshing out. To do that he had to maintain a zero-degree deck angle—keep the aircraft's nose pointed directly at the horizon—which pretty much ruled out a normal descent.

Edminster was at forty-one thousand feet and passing over Denver when he radioed air traffic control in San Antonio to ask if he could begin descending.

"Sir, you're three hundred fifty miles away from your airport."

"I know."

"And you want to start your descent now?"

"I do. A very slow three hundred to five hundred foot per minute descent if we could."

"What's the reason for this?"

Edminster, in his deep, steady voice: "I have a whale in the back."

You can imagine the silence on the other end of the radio.

San Antonio gave him the longest runway they had. He didn't use brakes when he touched down, just thrust reverse, and let the jet roll all the way to the end of the tarmac without spilling a drop. How steady could he fly this thing? That's how steady.

49

Dent wasn't yet in a panic but the idea of panicking had definitely entered the room. He was still searching for a runway to land his jet when the phone rang. He answered and the voice on the other end was plain and straightforward.

"Dent, it's John Nadeau. Sounds like we need to talk."

Nadeau was port director for US Customs and Border Protection at Bangor International Airport where 75 percent of Phoenix's foreign flights reentered the US and also the proposed landing site for the Ebola mission. Nadeau knew and trusted Phoenix, he liked Dent and got a kick out of what he considered the wild-ass spirit of the Phoenix crews who passed through his customs ramp carrying dangerous cargo of every imaginable stripe. That they used Bangor was a function of both its size and location. Bangor is quiet and out of the way, with a long, straight runway and little to no congestion. You can land anything there—NASA approved Bangor for shuttle landings. Nadeau sometimes told his neighbors that if they knew what was passing over their heads they wouldn't sleep at night. Now Dent was testing that reputation by trying to bring in Ebola.

"Can you describe to me how you're going to do it?"

Dent leaned back in his chair: "How much time you got?"

Nadeau listened as Dent went through the whole thing for him. Nadeau had been in Seattle after 9/11 and developed a protocol for inspecting the manifests of shipping containers entering the US from around the world. He was experienced, accustomed to intractable problems, and understood the basics of how a virus spreads. Not a lot, but enough. If the ABCS was designed for safely transporting an airborne disease, then he saw no reason why it couldn't safely transport Ebola. But he wanted to be sure.

When news of this plan was first being floated a couple days prior, Nadeau had spent a few hours flipping through the US Customs manuals. An aircraft inbound with dangerous cargo and broken landing gear—they had a plan for that. An aircraft inbound with an armed assailant onboard—they had a plan for that. But an aircraft carrying infectious disease—there was no plan. Fine, no plan. Nadeau reached out to his chain of command to say he saw no reason to prohibit the landing and asked if they had any guidance on how he should proceed. He heard nothing. So he called back.

"So what do we do," Nadeau asked his superiors in Washington. "Because I don't think we can say no."

Silence over the line.

"If he can't land here," Nadeau said, "then what? He dies over there? Okay, give me a name to put on that order." Nadeau stared at the speaker phone on his desk, daring it to answer. "Because it won't be mine."

He was told someone would get back to him with guidance, but now it was Friday and the aircraft was in the air and on the way, and still he hadn't heard a thing. It was like nobody in DC wanted to touch this thing, which surprised Nadeau but didn't shock him. He'd been in government long enough to know that when a problem comes along requiring the creative bending of rules, everyone with career aspirations goes into hiding. Nadeau was on an island. And that island only became more isolated when the local airport authority announced its intention to stop the flight from landing in Bangor.

So he reached out to Dent. And from everything he was hearing there was no risk to his customs crews on the ground, no risk to airport staff, certainly no risk to the city at large. And these were Americans they were talking about. He told Dent that he saw no reason not to help. Dent said that he'd gotten calls from state officials there warning that they would prohibit any plane carrying Ebola from landing at Bangor. What he wanted to know now was whether Nadeau had the resolve to stare them down.

"My customs circle is federal land, not state," Nadeau said. "I don't answer to them."

Dent smiled in relief: "That's all I need to hear."

With reentry taken care of, Dent rang up Walters and said he still needed a place to off-load the patient. The federal government doesn't have influence over civilian airports, but Walters told Dent to call Dobbins Air Reserve Base just outside of Atlanta. They might be game. A Phoenix Air dispatcher called and asked permission, then was told to wait while his request was passed up the chain of command. A few minutes later an airman came back over the line.

"It's denied. The colonel said not only no, but hell no."

As the sun rose over Bangor on Saturday morning, John Nadeau stood on the runway waiting. He'd arranged for the Gray Bird to land at a quiet spot tucked away from the camera crews who'd rushed up to Maine for footage of the arrival. At 8 a.m. aircraft N173PA landed. Nadeau stood by as it taxied to his customs ramp. Ebola was officially on US soil.

Dent sat in Cartersville willing his phone to ring. Where was Walters? Then dispatch yelled from outside that the jet had landed in Bangor for refuel and crew swap. It wouldn't be long now until they were back in the air and en route to Atlanta with a critical patient and nowhere to land.

Nadeau watched as his guys approached the jet. He knew they were anxious, but he trusted Phoenix Air and their ABCS, trusted Dent, and anyway none of them would be going anywhere near Ebola. All they had to do was collect the flight documents and passports, then wave the aircraft on with a smile. His guys didn't even have to board it. They would simply take Phoenix's word that whoever the paperwork claimed to be inside was in fact inside. This was a breach of protocol but not without precedent. All kinds of planes passed over Nadeau's ramp, most notably Air Force One—did anyone really think customs agents climbed aboard Air Force One and demanded to see the President of the United States? Exceptions were made.

Still. Ebola, liquifying bodies, zombies, and the end of the world—people were scared. He told his crew to wear whatever protective gear made them comfortable but cringed now as they approached the jet in full PPE. The suits sent a message to every airport employee within sight that this particular landing was so incredibly dangerous you needed head-to-toe protection just to witness it, something he feared would (and very quickly did) cause problems for him in Bangor.

A fuel truck backed up and connected its hose to the jet. Then the aircraft's fore door opened and out stepped Henry Hiteshew. This was a tense moment. Nobody on the ground wanted anything that'd been inside the aircraft coming out, but they needed to do a crew swap. Two new pilots—Jerry Haag and Brent Hardy—were getting on board to fly the final leg home, while pilot Brian Edminster hopped in the back and became a passenger. Hiteshew drew the short straw and would spend a lonely few days holed up in a Bangor hotel room waiting for the second flight carrying Nancy Writebol, on which he'd serve as relief for its crew. Nadeau did *not* want anyone to see Hiteshew getting off the airplane. The last thing he needed was panic inside Bangor International Airport because someone inside identified the man sitting next to him as the person who'd just climbed off the Ebola jet. He quickly ushered Hiteshew into the customs building, told him to change out of his flight gear and into civilian clothes, to slip quietly into the airport and act like nothing happened. To vanish. Hiteshew wasn't big on the idea of being all by himself and identified as the Ebola pilot, so he was only too happy to comply. A few minutes later, he was in the airport in jeans and a T-shirt standing alongside a scrum of news crews filming the Ebola plane. He watched for a bit and then he slipped unnoticed into the crowd.

Nadeau didn't watch the jet take off. He was already back inside the customs building compiling a detailed report for DC. Everything had gone well and his crew had performed exactly as expected. They had quickly and efficiently handled the first-ever Ebola flight into the US and he still hadn't heard anything from his superiors. As he typed up his report, he couldn't help wondering how it would be received and, more, what local reaction would be to news that not only had the first flight landed in their midst but that another was on the way.

Dent had secretly feared they wouldn't get approval to land at Dobbins. He and Walters from the very beginning had said over and over on every call they'd been on that Ebola was contained inside the patient, who'd be contained inside the ABCS, which was contained inside the aircraft. Containment. Technology. Multiple layers of protection. They staked a guarantee on their lives, on *every* American life, that Ebola wouldn't get off that airplane because no Ebola *patient* would get off that plane. Until now. This was the point in the mission where containment would have to be broken so the patient could be removed from the aircraft and driven across the full length of the base with nothing more sophisticated protecting everyone stationed there but the rolled-up windows of a municipal ambulance. Dent knew Walters had pull, that he was relentless, a bulldozer, that he could move mountains. But he couldn't begin to imagine how Walters would make this particular mountain budge. Then his phone rang. He snatched it off the cradle.

"Call again." It was Walters. Characteristically blunt. "Make a request for a permit and it should be granted."

Asked how he did it, Walters would say only that calls were made and the right thing was done. "People eventually come around to reason," is a characteristic Walters euphemism. What exactly happened to make the base commander come around to reason remained unsaid.

Again Dent called Dobbins Air Reserve Base and again he requested clearance to land. He was told by a man with a quivering voice that he needed to talk to the major. He was put on hold and then the major came on.

"Okay, we're going to let you land," the major said. "But you're not going to get any services. Fuel, nothing."

Dent was fine with that: "We don't need anything except to drop our door and we'll be gone." He did have one question, though. When his dispatcher had called earlier to get permission, it'd been a colonel who said no. Was the colonel good with this, and did they need to talk?

"The colonel won't talk to you; I'm talking to you," the major said.

Dent thanked the major, hung up, then yelled for dispatch to raise the Gray Bird on the radio. They finally had a place to land.

Edminster watched from his seat in the back as Haag and Hardy piloted the aircraft 1,300 miles from Bangor International to Atlanta and touched down at Dobbins a few minutes before noon on Saturday morning. During taxi, Jonathan turned on his phone to find a text from his oldest daughter saying there were people online making threats toward the crew for bringing Ebola back to the US. He texted back telling her not to worry, that it was just people talking, but he decided to check anyway. He immediately regretted it. Jonathan found posts online and even on his Facebook page saying Kent shouldn't be brought back and that everyone involved, Jonathan included, ought to be punished if anything went wrong. The volume and tenor of the comments was shocking, and he tried to put it out of his mind as he geared up to go in the ABCS to prep Kent for the transfer. But he couldn't shake it. More important, he was Kent, who'd nearly died halfway around the world and who now was probably just relieved to be home, to see his family. Jonathan wanted to prepare him for what was coming.

"Hey, uh, listen," he said as he changed Kent into a clean set of scrubs and PPE. "Most people appreciate everything you've done and want you to get better. But not everybody." Jonathan couldn't tell if this was sinking in with Kent or if he'd even remember it—looking at him now, Jonathan thought Kent's condition had worsened during transport. But he pressed on. Considering what he'd just seen, he worried there might be protestors at Emory (there were) and he wanted, in his own straightforward way, to ease Kent into it. "A lot of people aren't happy about us bringing you back to the US. You gotta just block out the negative, because there are some real assholes out there."

Vance and Doug draped the interior of the aircraft and then opened the door. The ambulance was waiting. It was time to break containment.

50

Gail Stallings should've been home sleeping or playing with her dogs or maybe, even if she's a little embarrassed to admit it, checking the matches on her dating profile. Anywhere but Dobbins. Gail grew up in Colorado, speaks in a straightforward voice that breaks unexpectedly into a high-pitched giggle, and in the summer of 2014 was a 9-1-1 paramedic in Atlanta. Medical emergencies in the city are handled not by firefighters but paramedics working for Grady Memorial Hospital, a massive public health system and one of only two Level 1 trauma centers in the state. Grady is underfunded and the staff is overworked, expected under impossible conditions to do everything for just about everyone living and dying on the long sweep of land between the North Georgia mountains and the Atlantic ocean. The place is hard on people. Surviving at Grady requires but also inspires the kind of fatalistic exuberance to say, *All this chaos isn't healthy but I can't live without it.* Picture a gunslinger fresh out of bullets who agrees to one more shootout. This outlook has made its way to Grady EMS.

In the 1990s a reticent Grady medic and Army veteran named Aaron Jamison started a tactical squad that was trained and equipped to accompany the SWAT team. Once Dr. Bruce Ribner had his Serious Communicable Diseases Unit up and running at Emory, the CDC approached Grady about handling the transports and Jamison's tactical squad became the Special Operations Team. The team trained alongside Ribner's doctors and nurses, dressing out to treat and transport mock patients suffering from various highly infectious diseases. Gail Stallings was a special ops medic, which meant when she wasn't at work she was on call in the event that something big dropped. Or that's how it had been until the spring of 2014 when the team was disbanded because someone decided that, like Ribner's lab at Emory, it hadn't been used enough to justify the expense. By the time efforts were underway to bring home two Americans fighting for their lives against Ebola, the only EMS providers capable of safely transporting them—the Grady EMS Special Operations Team—had already been mothballed.

With the team gone Gail had something new in her life—time to herself. It was her sister who'd talked her into the whole online dating thing. It wasn't Gail's personality, not really, not at first, but after being at it a couple months she had to admit it worked. She was meeting guys and going on dates, having fun. Even if she was still a little embarrassed about the whole thing, her sister had been right. Gail had plans that weekend but they got scratched on Friday when Jamison called out of the blue. He didn't provide much information, just said, "Hey come in, we're doing a thing."

Jamison, who goes by AJ, isn't really a talker and a line like that, from him, more or less constitutes oversharing. Gail had been working with AJ for years, appreciated his idiosyncrasies and knew by *doing a thing* he meant the team had been called up. "There is no thing," she said. "We don't have a team."

"We're doing a thing. State Department's involved. Get your ass in here."

Gail just nodded: "Okay."

She arrived at HQ with John Arevalo, the only other medic from the team still working at Grady. Arevalo is short with a tightly manicured beard—the kind of guy always in sunglasses, always smiling, and coolly placid. You cannot imagine him getting worked up. AJ—always with a cigarette, resigned as a solider and medic to a life of fixing other people's problems—was there when they arrived. So too was an observer from the State Department who told Gail and Arevalo that they, as the last remnants of Grady's Special Operations Team, were the only people trained and equipped to handle this transport. Gail just listened, the whole time thinking to herself *of course*. They'd been shut down right when they were needed most and now, like the punchline to some cosmic joke, the world was scrambling to re-create the capability it'd only recently deemed unnecessary. If you couldn't follow the thread between overconfidence and unpreparedness, then she couldn't help you. She stifled a laugh but couldn't hide the smirk. The world's a very funny place if you have the right kind of eyes.

The observer from State asked them to drag out their equipment and give him a full demonstration of how they'd handle the transport. "I want to watch you walk through it first," he said. "That goes well, you're going to take this person in."

It went well, they'd lost none of their edge in three months, and they were told to return at sunup the following morning for the real thing. AJ said not to show up at headquarters but instead report across the street where Grady kept an inconspicuous logistics building. Grady EMS had already been identified in the news as the agency most likely to transport the incoming Ebola patients. Gail wasn't sure of the details, and didn't ask, but AJ suggested there'd been death threats. He wanted to keep their names as far out of this story as he could.

"Just keep your heads down and your mouths shut," he said as they walked out the door.

That night Gail went home, ate dinner, and slept.

Or she tried to. There was too much going through her head. Little things, like did she drink enough water. It was going to be hot tomorrow, August in Georgia hot, and she'd be standing on a runway in a rubber suit. She got out of bed and drank a big glass of water. Then drank another. There was also excitement (just a little) and fear (not a ton) about what tomorrow would bring. She trusted her training and equipment, trusted Arevalo, and though she knew Ebola was harder to transmit than an airborne virus—which she'd transported once before—she also knew transmission was more likely in a confined space. The back of an ambulance is a textbook definition of confined space. Maybe it wasn't the longest night she'd ever pass, but it was long.

She was up early Saturday morning—dressed, showered, and out the door. She parked outside the logistics building and got to work. Gail and Arevalo checked and packed their PPE and medical gear, then tented the ambulance. Like Vance they used heavy-gauge plastic tarps to cover the bench seat, the captain's chair, all the cabinets and shelves, and even hung a tarp over the inside of the back door. They left only the stretcher and its floor mounts uncovered, everything else was enclosed in a white plastic shell. Gail and Arevalo were both experienced medics, they'd been on the team for years and had run God knows how many SWAT calls together, but this one was different. Somber almost, because of the risk to themselves, to Grady, the community. Everyone was watching them, even the State Department was watching. If something went wrong—and there are so many ways things can go wrong when you're driving a critical patient through a major urban area—the whole world would come down on their heads.

There was pressure and a little anxiety, maybe a lot of anxiety, and what are you going to do with that? Spend an hour dwelling on it, worrying, overthinking? If you've spent your adult life working on an ambulance, you're going to laugh. At the situation, at each other, at the fact that the world is surely doomed if the United States government has no one more qualified than *you* they can turn to in this moment. They talked trash the whole way up, hit Dobbins, and were escorted to a runway where they were told the aircraft was twenty minutes out. They quickly dressed—the same Tyvek suit, gloves, and mask that Phoenix was wearing except the Grady crew also had battery-powered respiratory devices, which were overkill, but their philosophy about PPE was that if you're going to be trapped in the back of an ambulance with a big, scary bug, you might as well level up.

As the aircraft appeared on the horizon everything

was set except for one detail—they hadn't decided who would drive and who would ride in the back with the patient. They quickly faced each other, left arm out, palm up, right hand balled into a fist—*one, two, three, shoot.* Arevalo won the rock, paper, scissors. Or lost, depending on how you see it. He'd ride in the back. Gail would drive.

Georgia in August is a miserable place. A sauna set on fire. The heat and humidity were worse at Dobbins because there was no escape from the sun and the tarmac was a frying pan. Gail stood melting into her PPE, all that rubber and plastic, panting into the respirator, as Arevalo disappeared inside the Gulfstream III. He emerged backward, holding onto Kent, along with a third person she didn't know, who was calling out the steps as he went. Kent flopped exhausted onto their stretcher. She couldn't help but sneak a glance as she leaned down to buckle him in. Here was the man whose illness had sparked an international rescue that set off panic and hysteria and anger, so much anger there was enough left over for her just because she was asked to help; a man whose efforts to save strangers was met at home with jeers, with calls to let him die, whose plight in the long run-up to the presidential election inspired a low-water mark in American decency.

Sensing in the moment exactly what Gail had sensed, Arevalo leaned over Kent and looked him square in the eye. "Welcome home."

This next part they'd done countless times but never in so fraught a situation. Gail's mind raced as they went through the intimate choreography of loading a critical patient into an ambulance. She'd seen all the ways things that *can* go wrong *do* go wrong, and all that experience was riding with her now. What if there's a problem while they're lifting the stretcher? What if he starts vomiting blood into his mask, or his PPE tears or her PPE tears? What if the stretcher locks up (it happens) or collapses (a lot)? *Plan for contingencies* is a phrase that lives in the back of every medic's mind because in critical situations they're always shorthanded. In the twenty minutes between the time they arrived and touchdown of the aircraft they discussed this, and they agreed to check in on each other, use eye contact, keep everybody level. Gail glanced up and there was Arevalo. Nothing said but it's all there in the look—it's just us. And we got this. She returned to the mantra that had carried her through every critical situation she faced on the street. *No running. Slow is smooth, smooth is fast. Steady. Just another day. Everything is everything.*

And it stayed with her as they loaded Kent into the plastic-shrouded cocoon of their ambulance, as she closed the door and made her way up front, as she put the truck in gear and drove off the base. That sense of serenity was there right up to the moment she turned out of Dobbins and straight into a mile-long gauntlet of media trucks, all lined up on both sides of the road. A single word escaped her lips as a hundred different cameras all swung to her at once:

"Fuck."

"Dent..." A voice from the hallway. "Turn on the television, you're not gonna believe this."

"What channel?"

The answer was any channel, all of them, it's the only news there was. The world had paused and stood in place, and from the silence burst a lone ambulance carrying the most famous patient on the planet. News helicopters filmed the whole thing from above, sharing airspace with police helicopters, which were in communication with cops on the ground. And they were only part of the contingent. The FBI was there as well, and this part caught even Walters by surprise. Like Dent he'd been focused on the air transport, but the bigger threat from a law enforcement standpoint was what would happen, or maybe even could happen, once Kent was out of the aircraft and on the ground. The FBI considered Ebola so dangerous they worried that terrorists might try to take advantage of its introduction to the US, that they might try to steal it and weaponize it or, more precisely, that they might try to weaponize Kent.

It sounded crazy, but so many threats had come in and were still coming, really this was just the beginning, that Walters coordinated with the FBI to have agents on the ground following the ambulance all the way from Dobbins to Emory, with air support for route recon. Even Grady had taken the step of outfitting a second ambulance in the event that one of the anonymous callers phoning in threats was serious and tried to sabotage the mission. It was total insanity.

Dent watched it all from his office. His television showed a split screen of the ambulance chase down I-75 on one half and on the other his own headquarters, beamed in from camera crews camped outside his window, the whole thing narrated by news anchors giving a surreal voiceover to the culmination of his life's work while hate trolls on the internet and on Twitter threw tantrums. It was *Fahrenheit 451* brought to life and updated for the twenty-first century. It was so real it wasn't real at all.

And there was Gail Stallings. Behind the wheel of the ambulance wearing a Tyvek suit, non-latex nitrile gloves, and an N95 mask, cameras zoomed in on her face, her partner in the back with a highly contagious patient, and the whole world watching. She was just trying to keep it between the lines. She knew that most people had tricked themselves into thinking they were safe, that an ocean and technology and the privilege of being American would protect them from the contagions plaguing the rest of the world. That many people refused to accept that the arrival of a virus on our shores had always been a *when* not an *if*. She expected some craziness. But *this*? This was crazy on a whole other level. She maneuvered her way through the gauntlet of cameras at the front entrance of Dobbins, then beelined for the highway, and hit the onramp at speed. There were cop cars, unmarked FBI cars, helicopters overhead and buzzing around, chaos everywhere, but she trained her eyes on the road. News footage showed a driver coolly focused on driving, but not captured on film were her inner thoughts, which were significantly less cool and could be summed up as a rolling commentary of expletives.

She was speeding down the highway at seventy miles an hour with a patient the public viewed as a dirty bomb in the back of her ambulance and all she could think about was everything that could go wrong. She could have engine trouble or a flat tire, an accident even. *Holy hell, can you imagine an accident?* It was daytime, traffic everywhere, anything could happen. She needed to focus, to tune out the noise, and just drive. The words running repeatedly through her head were *Don't fuck this up, Stallings.*

It's thirty minutes from Dobbins to Emory, and a half hour is a long time to sit gripping the wheel. She was so intent on blocking out the noise, on keeping her eyes glued to the road, that she didn't see the car creeping toward them until it was almost in their lane. It came from nowhere, just appeared beside her. Crowded the dotted line and started swerving. She glanced over. The driver was leaning out his window, not looking at the road, camera out and filming. Gail was in the left lane, nowhere to go if he came any closer but into the concrete median, and this guy's not even driving anymore, he's just recording. It would have been almost funny if it hadn't been scary, if she hadn't been told about the death threats, if people weren't lining up to watch her pass, if the whole thing wasn't being broadcast live. As it was, she didn't know what the guy wanted or what he'd do. Was this the thing they'd all feared? It was definitely something she feared. He followed for a while, filming, until the cops swept in and chased him away.

Twenty minutes in they got off the highway, and now the whole convoy squeezed into narrow side streets. Helicopters and cops and the ambulance, lights and sirens, all barreling through neighborhoods, houses trembling from the end-times roar. Ribner and his staff were watching the procession on TV, thinking what everyone else was thinking—it's just like the OJ chase—except this time the circus was coming to him. When the wail of sirens outside got louder than the wail of sirens on TV and the helicopters started beating the air outside his window, he knew the moment had arrived. They were here.

51

Darrin Benton walked into his parents' house and found the front room empty. He called out, got no answer, and followed the sound of the television into the kitchen. His mother stood there in silence. He walked over next to her, she touched his arm without looking, and together the two of them watched the Gray Bird touch down at Dobbins. They looked on in awe like everyone else as the ambulance carrying the Ebola doctor raced through Atlanta. Darrin's mother turned to him as the ambulance reached Emory University Hospital and said, "You wouldn't do that, would you?"

The better question when it came to Darrin was what wouldn't he do. When he first applied to Phoenix they weren't hiring anyone to fly planes so instead he took a job washing them. Spent his first few months cleaning bathrooms. Eventually he earned a copilot's slot and since then he'd been all over the world. He'd flown medevacs out of the Caribbean as hurricanes made landfall, was not-so-briefly detained in Mali over confusion about his landing permit, and once spent a long and uneasy night in Peru sleeping aboard an aircraft packed full of hand grenades. He had girlfriends who couldn't deal with the schedule or the danger, and they'd say "It's either me or Phoenix." And he'd almost think about hanging it up, but then he'd be crossing the Pacific at night with the cockpit lights out, surrounded by nothing but stars, like outer space, and he'd be single by the time he landed. When his mother asked if he was willing to fly Ebola patients, he didn't have to think before answering.

"Heck yeah, I'd do that." His eyes were locked on the screen. "If we do another, I hope they call me for it."

Gail pulled the ambulance around the back of Emory and put it in park. She yelled back to Arevalo before getting out. They'd been here before for drills and knew what lay ahead. Ribner was a firm believer in keeping patients with highly infectious diseases as far from the main hospital as possible to avoid even the appearance of exposure. It's why the Serious Communicable Diseases Unit was tucked away in a far corner and also why Arevalo and Gail were effectively bringing Kent to the back door. Between their ambulance and the unit lay a minefield of chunky rocks, a small concrete pad, the outer door, a corner too tight to negotiate with a stretcher, a steep set of stairs, and then another tight turn. Really, it wasn't a feasible entrance. Gail and Arevalo discussed between themselves the possibility of carrying Kent inside, but due to all the obstructions and their suits, the impossibility of clear communication between them, the cameras, it seemed too big a risk. They could easily fall and drop Kent, which felt, other than one of them getting exposed, like the second worst thing that could happen.

Arevalo turned to Kent. "Do you think you can walk into the hospital?"

Kent nodded. "Okay."

Arevalo opened the back door of the ambulance and stepped out. News cameras inside a hovering chopper zoomed in, anchors talked.

"Someone's getting out—"

"Do you think that's the doctor?"

"Surely, they sent a decoy. I'm sure he's coming in a different way."

Gail stayed in the ambulance. The place was a zoo. News trucks with their satellites and massive retractable antennas ringed the building. Dotted among them were reporters with microphones talking into cameras on tripods. Helicopters buzzed overhead. There wasn't a parking space or patch of open grass within a half mile of the hospital. The international media swarmed

Emory like ants on a lollipop. The rest of the hospital's staff had yet to weigh in but uncertainty among them—fed by a steady stream of fear and invective from the outside world—was growing.

"If this genie is released from its bottle and unleashed here in Georgia there is no turning back!" This from a commenter to a story about the rescues printed in the *Atlanta Journal-Constitution*. "The Potential of Deaths in the Millions are to be expected. A fence will be erected all around Atlanta and there will be NO coming in or coming OUT!" In another forum, one man wondered why scientists were letting "these Trojan horses, these lepers, into our midst."

Emory responded to the noise by posting armed guards around the hospital entrances. The city sent a police canine unit to sniff the perimeter for bombs. But there was no such protection for Gail. It'd been a strange morning, and she was spent. As soon as Arevalo had transferred Kent and emerged from the hospital, she put the truck in gear and sped off. She'd been sweating for hours and just wanted to go home and rest. The next patient, due in only a couple days, would be hers.

It hadn't been five minutes when Darrin's phone rang. It was the Phoenix dispatcher.

"We have another flight leaving tomorrow and we'd like you on it."

"You got it."

Click. It really was that fast. One minute he was watching his coworkers make history and the next he was part of it. Darrin was still in the kitchen, still standing next to his mother. The news was still beaming back images from Emory Hospital, reporters still talking about hemorrhagic fevers and outbreaks and fatality rates, how Ebola would thrive in the confined spaces of an airplane or ambulance. But it all looked different now. Tomorrow it would be him on that plane. This was really happening. He got hit with a flood of jitters, of adrenaline, of the thousand things he needed to do before morning. Darrin looked over at his mom and saw she had tears in her eyes. She grabbed his arm and asked if he was sure about this. Because she wasn't, she didn't like the idea at all.

"Mom, this is what I do."

She nodded and straightened up. Patted his arm. "Then we need to get everybody together, whole family. I'll make buttermilk pie."

"Mom..."

She was firm. "If you're going to do this, we're all having dinner."

Darrin tried to protest but there was no getting out of it. If he was flying into the middle of an Ebola outbreak, then she was throwing him a Last Supper. His mom called each of her three sisters, called Darrin's sister, called their extended family and family friends, everyone, told them all that Darrin was now in the middle of this Ebola stuff and to be there, no excuses, for dinner because, well, because you never know.

While his family planned out his last meal, Darrin jumped in his car and went to get ready. He'd just gotten back from a medical flight to Japan and hadn't been to his house in a week. He had to drop off laundry, pick up dry cleaning, and pack for Liberia, all before the crew got back to Cartersville. He wanted to be there when they landed, to talk to them and glean whatever information he could about the upcoming flight. He pressed harder on the gas. And all the while his phone kept ringing. His sister, his friends, family he hadn't seen in a while—they all wanted to know if he was really going to Liberia and why. Did he really want to put himself at risk like that? Everyone he talked to seemed nervous and unsettled, and even though most were supportive, he just couldn't keep having the same conversation. He decided to stop answering and let everything go to voicemail. The minute he decided no more calls, his phone rang with the one call he couldn't ignore. The screen flashed a single, magical name. Wendy.

Wendy, whom he met that summer on a fishing trip

to Alaska. Wendy who was beautiful and funny and liked sports and fishing and who, despite her resistance to being set up by Mark Thompson, eventually warmed to Darrin and kissed him on the flight home. Wendy who was perfect and out of his league and yet somehow still interested in Darrin, or was anyway, until he scared her off by sending a dozen roses to her house immediately after they got back to Atlanta. Wendy, who broke it off, who said she wasn't ready for a relationship, and hadn't spoken to him in weeks. Wendy. Darrin picked up.

"Mark called," she said with a hint of concern but also intrigue in her voice. "He said you're going to Africa tomorrow and might not come back." Darrin shook his head—frigging Mark. Wendy paused, then: "You want to have dinner?"

52

Speculation about how doctors would save Kent began the instant he disappeared inside Emory. Little was known, even among infectious disease experts, about treating Ebola other than, in West Africa, a diagnosis was something just this side of receiving a death sentence. In the popular imagination, anyone with something so deadly and communicable, so absolutely terrifying, would be treated inside an advanced government facility with alarms and airlocks, maybe even with guards posted and ready to kill anyone who tried to break out. The mind goes to Michael Crichton, it goes to *The Andromeda Strain*, where a team of specialists is whisked off to a secret underground facility programmed to self-destruct unless they can identify the pathogen and devise a cure. This particular building in Atlanta might not self-destruct, but Kent Brantly had been transported across the globe to a renowned research hospital with longstanding ties to the Centers for Disease Control and Prevention, and would now be treated inside a Serious Communicable Diseases Unit by experts in infectious disease. After the chaos of the transport you could be forgiven, once the steel door slammed shut, if you expected futuristic technology and science fiction, if in your mind what awaited Kent at the top of that narrow flight of stairs was God himself, called down by the government to save the human race.

What Kent got was Bruce Ribner. Salt-and-pepper hair, stylish glasses, serious in that doctor-y way but also self-effacing and funny. Ribner wasn't interested in the science fiction or pop culture versions of Ebola, nor did he care about the rantings of people who wanted him to stop—though he didn't yet know how crazy it was about to get. He was curious about, but put little stock in, experimental treatments. He didn't have magic protocols. What he had were dedicated professionals, most of them nurses, capable and willing to provide around-the-clock ICU care to every patient who entered the unit. Starting with Kent Brantly.

Kent had miraculously been able to walk into the unit, but it was immediately clear to Ribner that he was deathly ill and required aggressive treatment. Whether he survived depended largely on his body's natural defenses—it would be Ribner's job to keep Kent alive long enough for the body to fight the virus.

They needed to get Kent connected to heart and oxygen monitors, they needed to start IV lines and also to draw blood so a full panel of labs could be run. His body chemistry and organ function were concerning unknowns.

Even before the blood work came back, Ribner had indications of what he was up against. A 12-lead EKG takes readings of the heart's electrical activity from several different angles, and Ribner described what he saw on the monitor as hideous. The culprit was a dangerously low potassium level caused by extreme and pronounced dehydration from a week of hemorrhaging, vomiting, diarrhea, and sweating. Potassium is necessary for muscle contractions, nerve and kidney function, and the regulation of the heartbeat and blood pressure. Even moderately low potassium levels can disrupt all this. Severe depletion leads to kidney failure, respiratory paralysis, and deadly cardiac arrythmias—precisely what Ribner spotted on Kent's EKG. Getting potassium in the patient was step one, though the blood panel, once it was in, might reveal other, even more concerning problems. Blood chemistries veering wildly from the norm are evidence of a vicious, internal assault on the body. How long any one individual can withstand the assault is dependent on too many different factors to accurately predict outcomes. Who lives and who dies can seem at times to rest on the whims of fate. Ribner did not plan on leaving Kent's fate to chance.

His blood was frequently drawn, he was constantly monitored, forever prodded. It was unending treatment, all of it intimate and hands-on, requiring close contact with Kent and the handling of dirty linen, equipment, and needles. Every movement was heightened by the need to be careful, by a personal and collective policing of safety and protocols. Because Kent was a healthcare worker everyone in the unit was also experiencing, like Linda Mobula before them, an added sense of responsibility leavened by a *this-could've-been-me* gravity. It was stressful and daunting but Ribner was acutely aware that as the first facility to receive an Ebola patient evacuated from a hot zone, the unit had the opportunity to set an example for the rest of the world. One way or another they were going to prove just how safe this really was.

Between the risks and the stakes, the continued media attention, the growing rumbles of discontent—even from within the hospital itself—Ribner, in typically understated fashion, told anyone who asked that it was "a pretty exciting time."

53

The whole thing with Wendy almost never happened. Mark Thompson had planned a trip to Alaska with a girl he was dating and she wanted to bring her friend, someone named Wendy, and Mark thought it would make everything easier if he too brought a friend along, someone he could set this Wendy up with, to even out the numbers. Mark dragged Darrin Benton to Alaska but failed to mention that this girl, whom Darrin had never met, didn't know she was being set up and definitely didn't sound like the type who'd appreciate it. Which didn't stop Mark from trying. The whole week he found ways to force Darrin and Wendy together, devised one artificial situation after another, each more obvious than the last. And the harder Mark tried the harder Wendy fought it. Mark Thompson, who's not known for quitting or for his subtlety, kept at it until finally Darrin had to pull Wendy aside and explain that he wasn't behind the setup and that he was just as uncomfortable as she was. She didn't buy it. And yet, eventually, they bonded. They had a couple good days in Alaska, then the flight home and the kiss and everything seemed great until Darrin sent the flowers and completely ruined it. For weeks he'd been hoping she would call (she never did) and now here she was, unexpectedly inviting him to dinner because Mark—of course it was Mark—had told her that Darrin was off to do something dangerous and that it was probably his last night on Earth.

Classic Mark. This time Darrin didn't resist. Whatever Wendy felt about him, he was wild about her and thought that maybe, if given a chance, this might turn into something. He said yes to dinner almost before she finished asking. He hung up, kept driving, almost forgot where he was going. The last hour had been madness and into that swirl of competing emotions he added one more, guilt. Darrin drove back to his parents' house. His mom was still working the phones, still making plans. He walked her out back, put his arm over her shoulder. He's close with his family, the middle child, a bit of a mama's boy. But there was something special about his stalled relationship and he didn't want to miss this chance to revive it.

"You remember that girl I met? She called..."

His mother knew, they always know, and she gave

him a look like *you gotta be kidding me*. But she sighed and hugged him. Smiled. "It's okay. Go."

A few minutes later his aunts began to arrive. Darrin Benton was the only person in his family not there for his own Last Supper.

54

The Gray Bird arrived back in Cartersville at 2:15 p.m. on Saturday afternoon and was towed to the maintenance hangar where it would sit under the armed guard of a Bartow County Sheriff's Office deputy. Between now and the next flight a long list of critical things needed to happen, including decon. Conversations during the development of the ABCS between the CDC and Phoenix had touched on decontamination but never got into specifics. Phoenix always assumed, since they had no experience in, or equipment for, decontaminating infected surfaces, that this would be handled by the CDC. But the CDC had no such intentions. They sent advisors and chemicals to Phoenix but they were not getting on that plane.

Doug, Vance, and Jonathan all stared at each other in disbelief. Kent had spent more than twelve hours in the tent, the whole thing was full of contaminated PPE, contaminated equipment, and contaminated surfaces. It was wall-to-wall Ebola. Vance had been awake for days, sweating and training and worrying, exposing himself to a frightful contagion while caring for an incredibly sick patient and just when he thought he'd made it out to the other side—he'd already changed into regular clothes—the CDC team was telling him he had to go back and do more. He felt his soul leave his body and evaporate in the stifling air of the hangar. He didn't want to do it. He *really* didn't want to do it.

But it had to be done. As the senior people, he and Doug volunteered. They climbed back into PPE as the CDC team gave them sprayers and instructions. Doug and Vance trudged into the ABCS and for nearly two hours they sprayed down every surface and piece of equipment. Vance sweated the whole time. Sweated through his shoes and his belt, both of which he had to throw away. Sweated himself out too—by the time he was done he'd lost three pounds. Then they limped away to get some rest, but only a little. They'd be back tomorrow to do it all over again. Nancy Writebol still needed to come home.

55

Despite having gotten two doses of ZMapp, Nancy was still bedridden. Her condition could be guessed at but remained unknown because unlike Ribner at Emory, Linda wasn't able to run a 12-lead EKG or send off blood samples. She had no way of knowing just how dangerously low Nancy's potassium levels were. But she knew her patient was still very much in trouble. And so did Nancy's husband David. He woke each day, shrugged clumsily into his PPE, and sat by his wife's side not knowing each time he entered if this day would be her last. To make his time count, because who knows, he sat on her bed and they talked, and when she couldn't respond he talked enough for both of them. Her life so obviously hung in the balance that neither shied from the subject. They had discussions, hard discussions, about what would happen if she died. Rescue, though still uncertain, was at least being attempted. Salvage was a whole other question. In fact, it wasn't even a question; it was a given. If she died now, her body—no longer a vessel for the human soul but simply a vector for deadly pathogens—would be buried here in Liberia. Nancy and David spoke about where and how a local burial would happen. These were serious conversations, frank and practical, but also loving. There was no question in either of their minds that David would do anything for Nancy, so why not work out the details now. For Nancy, bedridden and deathly ill, David's presence felt something like grace. For Linda, a witness to all this, it was more complicated.

When Nancy became sick, David pulled Linda aside and said, "I really love my wife and I would walk through fire for her." He wanted Nancy's caregivers to feel the same. Linda was just barely in her thirties and relatively new to medicine. She had treated the sick and dying in dangerous places but never under such intimate and unrelenting conditions. The work had taken its toll and pushed her to the edge of what she could endure. Nancy was due to be evacuated in two days. Linda could only hope the first trip had gone well, that America received and accepted Kent and was ready for Nancy because she wasn't sure how much longer she could last.

56

There would be no more Ebola flights through Bangor International Airport. Port Director John Nadeau had naively and possibly even mistakenly allowed the first to land, but surely he'd learned his lesson. That was the prevailing sentiment in Maine, a state unaccustomed to the spotlight, so when Nadeau made clear he'd already approved another flight, due to land in under forty-eight hours, the feeling that came back to him was *Holy shit, you haven't learned your lesson?!* Things became uncomfortable.

It started with the airport employees, some of whom wore hazmat suits if they needed to enter or even just pass by the customs ramp. Fear spread and then came frustration—why was he letting this stuff in—and soon they were openly complaining. Because the airport is funded by both the local and state government, those complaints quickly made their way to officials only too happy to aim their frustration at Nadeau. He got angry calls from the offices of US Senator Susan

Collins and Governor Paul LePage demanding to know what he was doing and why. They told him to stop the flights (something he'd never allow) or else reroute them through Canada (something the Canadians would never allow). He was making enemies across half the state—a growing list of people wanted to burn him at the stake—and the second flight was still days away.

An emergency meeting was called at the airport to discuss the flights. Nadeau walked in and found himself staring down city and state public health officials, members of the airport authority, representatives from the City of Bangor, from the governor's office, and also from the offices of Senator Collins and Senator Angus King. The air was charged with fear and anger, much of it directed toward him. Nadeau sat and listened, he wanted to hear them out, and some of the conversation was about how the flights could be handled in a safe way so nothing broke out in the state, but most of what he heard was *Don't do this*.

He stood and spoke. He laid out the circumstances of the first flight, talked about how Kent was a fellow American, a doctor who'd gotten sick and needed to get home. He talked about the ABCS and how Kent posed no threat to the people of Maine.

"I don't see the risk," he said. "And I'm not blowing you off but what are you gonna do? That aircraft's coming in from the Azores and can only fly around so long before it runs out of fuel. Are we just going to let it crash?" He held up his hands. "Because that seems like a bad option to me."

People weren't happy with him, with the flights, with any of it. But Nadeau decided he'd heard enough from the state and wasn't going to listen anymore. The facts as he saw them were simple. He had a job to do and as a federal employee he didn't have to listen to the governor. The senate staffers were a different story. They didn't have the power to stop him but they could, if they wanted, make his life miserable. He'd hoped it wouldn't come to this, that someone above him would step up and take a little of the heat off him, but he still hadn't heard anything from DC. He walked out determined to assist the rescue, but an uneasy feeling was growing in his stomach. He had absolutely no backup. If anything went wrong, his career was over.

57

The modified Gulfstream III stood idle in the hangar. Before a second flight could launch a new ABCS tent needed to be installed and connected to the monitors, equipment, and filters. The reversed airflow system had to be turned on and tested, and the aircraft tuned, fueled, and readied for flight. This required a small army of workers swarming over every inch of the airplane. But the first step was to remove the old tent, which absolutely no one wanted to do.

Dent and Dr. Mike had tried to calm everyone's nerves, to answer whatever questions they had—*reassure* was a word Dent had used a lot. But among the maintenance crews and their families there was some hesitation about climbing inside the tent—still dripping disinfectant—and unfastening the hundreds of ties that connected it to the frame. That alone would take hours. And yeah, Dr. Mike said it was safe but there were doctors on television saying the opposite. So who were they supposed to believe? And anyway,

Vance and Doug didn't know anything about decontamination, they admitted as much, were forced into doing it really, which they had, but had they done it *right*? What if they hadn't, what if there was still Ebola in the tent, and what if they got it? It can take up to twenty-one days before symptoms start and were they supposed to quarantine from their families and friends, their jobs, their lives, for three weeks? The tent needed to come down, had to be packed up and shipped off to an incinerator in Florida, the whole maintenance department knew that. It had to be replaced so another mission to Liberia could be launched. But did that mean they had to be the ones who did it?

A group of guys not terribly eager to get within a hundred feet of the aircraft stood weighing their options as a call went up for volunteers to climb inside and deal with the tent. Quiet, hands not going up, everybody waiting, and into that silence two voices called out. Chris Allen, the airframe and powerplant mechanic who'd insisted on tinkering with the air filters until not a single part per million of infectious pathogen escaped them, stepped forward. Standing next to him was Tawn Heater. If Chris represented an understanding of the equipment and the process, Tawn embodied trust in the science.

Tawn was born in Miami and moved around but grew up mostly in Florida. When she was twelve her father died of a heart attack, one of those powerful and unexpected blows that sends you off in search of either refuge or answers. Tawn, always mechanically inclined, wanted to know why. She studied science and medicine, illness, disease, and pathology; the ways and reasons bodies wear down and fail. But only on the side, as a hobby, just one more thing that made her peculiar in a room full of aircraft mechanics. Tawn joined the Navy in the early '90s, the Clinton years, when the military was rethinking the sort of roles women could play in its ranks. She came on as an F-18 mechanic, one of the first females to be stationed on an aircraft carrier. Men lost their minds. She developed thick skin, got used to shit talk, and by the time she joined Phoenix in 2000 it hardly registered that she was the only woman in the hangar. A few years later she helped create Phoenix's Quality Assurance department, and it was there that she became involved in the development of the ABCS.

She knew the tent, knew viruses and infectious disease, and was comfortable enough to go inside. Tawn and Chris put on gloves then walked across the hangar toward the Gray Bird, the other mechanics watching, waiting to see if maybe they'd explode on contact or turn into zombies. They climbed the stairs to nervous laughter from below, to people saying, *You're gonna be bleeding out of your orifices*—the shit talk never stops.

It was humid inside and stuffy. Tawn was married and had a daughter at home and her family was on her mind as she bent to step inside the antechamber. The chemicals Doug and Vance had used to decontaminate the tent dripped from the ceiling and burned, like her skin was on fire. Tawn turned to Chris as they started undoing the ties and said, "Nothing's going to survive in here, not with this stuff."

On the other side of the runway, where the pilots gathered, Darrin Benton talked to Brian Edminster about the flight and Monrovia, about the hotel, about how Edminster had gone stalking through the airport in search of someone to approve his flight plans and give him clearance to take off. About the issues surrounding the landings at both Bangor and Dobbins. Darrin more or less felt ready for the mission as he left the airfield. A few miles away his family was gathering for his Last Supper, but Darrin jumped on the highway and drove south into the city to meet Wendy. They went to a steakhouse in Buckhead, ate dinner, drank wine, danced. They talked about the trip but not too much and eventually went back to her place. Darrin was still awake when the sun rose. Thinking about the flight. About walking through a hot zone in the middle of an outbreak. About whether last night meant he and Wendy could be getting back together for real.

He got out of bed at 8:30 a.m., searched Wendy's kitchen for coffee, brewed a pot, and stood watching the news. Almost twenty-four hours later and all they talked about was the flights. Wendy walked out, stood next to him in silence for a few minutes. Then, walking away: "Whole world's watching. Don't fuck this up."

58

Amber Brantly picked up the intercom telephone and said hello. The voice that came back was weak but familiar. Nothing separated her from Kent but the thick protective glass covering the window to his room. Kent was close now, closer than it seemed at times he'd ever get, but he still had so far to go.

It'd been a long two weeks. They were last together in Monrovia, before Ebola upended their lives. Amber was in Texas when the world finally took note of what was happening in West Africa, sitting in her parents' house, praying for good news but listening over the phone as Kent drifted into the ocean of disease and slowly started to sink. But then word of a rescue. She flew with Kent's parents and sister to Atlanta only to be told her own life was also in danger. The people who didn't want her husband here, who wanted him left to die overseas, American or not, those same people who were a threat to Kent and anyone treating him were also a threat to his family.

She checked into a hotel under the assumed name of Becky Woodall. She had the protection of a security detail headed by a former Secret Service agent named Tim Viertel, an absolute bear of a man who, camouflaged in a suit, looked like any other morning commuter on the Bethesda to DC rail line. Amber called Emory as soon as she arrived in Atlanta and was told Kent would have to be received, evaluated, and stabilized before anyone could see him. But it'd been two weeks of wondering if she'd have to listen to her husband die over the telephone and there was only so much more waiting she could take. She stood in her hotel room watching the landing and Kent's arrival at the hospital, and that's all she had to see. She called Tim.

"He's here—let's go!"

The whole group poured out of the hotel room and into the hallway where Tim was waiting to whisk them through the back door and into a pair of waiting Suburbans. Security was tight at Emory; Ebola hysteria was in full swing—reporters and media trucks everywhere, protestors lined up and shouting from the sidewalk. There didn't seem to be a way to get in unnoticed, but of course Tim had planned for this. Hospital security ushered them around the madness to a side entrance, then down a set of stairs and into the labyrinth of tunnels running beneath the hospital. Underground and unseen, rushing through dimly lit corridors, Amber eager to get there already and then, finally, arrival. The Serious Communicable Diseases Unit. Bruce Ribner met her at the entrance. He was optimistic but cautious, knew she'd watched Kent walk from the ambulance, and wanted to set expectations right away.

He looked at Amber and then in a direct but gentle voice said, "He's not out of the woods yet."

The unit had two patient rooms, both sealed off, that faced each other and were separated by a narrow waiting area. There was an intercom phone for each room and a viewing window, and looking through it now Amber saw Kent for the first time since this started. She felt relief in seeing him but fear too. Kent was swollen and puffy, his eyes were bloodshot. He was alive, yes, but incredibly sick and it showed. It's the hemorrhaging with Ebola that captures the imagination, but more often what kills you is the diarrhea, the constant gushing of fluids, all of them, into a diaper. It's death by humiliation, by torment. His fever was 102 degrees, his heart rate a rapid and unsustainable 120 bpm. The virus had assaulted his liver so badly for so long that he now had hepatitis, a condition made worse by all the Tylenol he'd been taking to stave off the fever—two extra-strength tabs every six hours since it started. His sodium, potassium, and albumin levels were all within fatal limits. Though he'd barely eaten in over a week and had been losing fluid at catastrophic levels, he hadn't lost an ounce of weight because of all the swelling. Kent was home, the first patient ever to be treated in the unit—first Ebola patient ever treated in the US—yet what he felt was not relief so much as trepidation. He'd seen Ebola kill too many people.

Amber felt it too. Kent still needed to receive the final two doses of ZMapp and maybe it would help—Ribner was unconvinced—but the very idea of experimental medicine made her incredibly nervous. That his survival remained uncertain was something she tried to push from her voice as she lifted the intercom phone.

She put her hand on the glass. "How was your trip?"

Kent said, "It was a trip."

"We watched you walk off the ambulance."

Kent, confused, looked back from his bed. "You were watching me?"

She smiled through tears. "The whole world was watching you."

This was true and not everyone was happy. A phone rang in the unit. Ribner answered. It was the chief nurse. She reached out several times a day to talk through progress but more often it was a problem she called about and she had one of those now.

Ribner began his medical career in the 1970s, peace time for epidemiologists, a decade when infectious disease experts were beginning to wonder if antibiotics and inoculations had forever cured us of deadly pathogens. Then came the 1980s and AIDS and that hope was exposed for the delicate thread it'd been. Ribner was working in Houston when the outbreak began, and he watched public reaction shift from alarm and confusion to full-blown panic. Truly concerning was the reaction among the medical community. No one knew what the disease was or where it came from, not until 1984 when HIV was listed as the likely cause. But it remained a death sentence, and as AIDS spread so did reluctance to treat it. Patients were either hidden away or else refused admission entirely, anything to keep from having to touch them. Ribner once got into a screaming match with the head of his hospital's orthopedic surgery department because she flatly refused to allow her surgeons to operate on any patient testing positive for HIV.

Over time AIDS hysteria only got worse. In July 1985 the actor and Hollywood icon Rock Hudson collapsed at the Ritz-Carlton in Paris. He was rushed unresponsive and near-death from his hotel to the American Hospital. The international press laid siege to the building and the world became riveted as reports surfaced that Hudson wasn't suffering from inoperable cancer as initially believed, but from AIDS. Hudson had starred in dozens of movies, shared the screen with

James Dean and Elizabeth Taylor, counted Ronald and Nancy Reagan as personal friends, but now, dying in Paris, his life was reduced to four scarlet letters. The hospital, which initially agreed to treat him, wilted under the attention. They now wanted him out. Hudson was flown to the US and died soon after, alone, in Los Angeles.

Here it was thirty years later and the world had changed entirely but also not at all. There was a new outbreak, a different besieged patient, but the rising tide of panic was exactly the same. And once again it was seeping into Ribner's hospital. And so this call from the chief nurse.

"I just a got a very interesting phone call from the staff upstairs," she told him. "They want to know if we can keep the cafeteria open later at night."

Ribner wasn't sure where this was going. "And why is that?"

"They can't have food delivered," she said. "Drivers refuse to enter Emory because they're afraid of Ebola."

And not just some delivery drivers but all delivery drivers. No tip was big enough to deliver pizza or Chinese to phlebotomy; there'd be no burritos for the anesthesiologists up in surgery. And it wasn't just that people refused to enter the hospital—they wanted anyone who'd been in there to stay as far from them as possible. Local restaurants hung signs in their windows that said *No Emory Employees Welcome Here.* Doctors couldn't drop their kids off at school without being accused of contaminating the entire campus. Then there were the picketers outside Emory with their chants and signs and expletives, whole lines of them that employees had to slip past just to get to work in the morning. And don't forget the mail. Thousands of packages addressed to the staff of the unit arrived every day, many of them anonymous and containing who knew what. CDC Director Tom Friedan was getting death threats, and right next door at Emory all those packages from unknown senders just kept piling up. The hospital established a temporary post office down the street just to receive them. Nothing was opened on-site, everything was scanned and x-rayed to make sure the suspicious package from Dallas or Reno or Coeur d'Alene, Idaho, wasn't a bomb.

Ribner wasn't prepared for this. An environment that just yesterday felt challenging but dynamic, today seemed crazy. He expected chaos but not how quickly chaos would curdle into fear. And all the while, the talking heads and politicians who'd come out against the transports kept turning up the pressure. It wasn't enough anymore to say Kent should be left to die in Liberia or that he'd gotten what he deserved. Now that he was here the focus shifted to Emory, to how unprepared they were, how they had no business treating

Ebola, how they were going to kill us all. The claims got weird: like that rats in the sewer system would come into contact with Ebola-tainted wastewater from the unit and those rats, carrying the disease, would rush out into the streets and start an outbreak in Atlanta. *It's plague times!* The Infowars website, run by conspiracy theorist Alex Jones, the guy who'd been insisting the CDC would someday create a pandemic just so the government could institute authoritarian rule, ran an article under the headline "Feds would exercise draconian emergency powers if Ebola hits US."

In that sense Ebola had already spread beyond the unit. So many people were predicting disaster that employees from other floors began wondering out loud just what exactly Ribner and his staff were doing down there in that far-off corner of the hospital. Maybe it wasn't such a good idea. Maybe it wasn't safe. Maybe everyone should stop coming to work until all this blew over. What started out as quiet dissent among hospital staff was beginning to resemble mutiny. Ribner was forced to turn his attention from the unit and Kent Brantly toward staff from the hospital at large. He set up a one-hour information session, the first of what would turn out to be many, in the auditorium for anyone with questions. Five hundred people showed up. They were terrified by what they'd been hearing and wanted to know what Ribner was doing to keep them safe. Like Dr. Mike before him, he went through the science, the safety measures, the fourteen years of training he'd done with the CDC, the fact that he wouldn't be doing this at all if he didn't think he could. There was no comingling of patients, he'd made sure of that. Nobody in the ICU or OB or a single surgical tech was going to get sick from what was happening in the unit. Despite what they were hearing elsewhere, he said, it was safe. And it was the right thing to do.

That sense of service and compassion might've resonated inside the walls of the health system, but outside no one wanted to hear it. Outside people seemed to feel that doing the right thing was fine just so long as they weren't the ones being asked to do it. As one online commenter posted, "The road to hell is paved with good intentions."

59

"Goddamn it!"

Henry Hiteshew didn't look. He was in Bangor eating lunch at a bar overlooking the Penobscot River and trying his best not to draw attention. He'd been left behind in Maine as relief for the crew that'd be coming in with Nancy Writebol, and now he was surrounded by locals who weren't at all happy their city was the point of entry for Ebola patients. For the most part he never left his hotel room. That's where he was when he watched the landing in Atlanta, with the news trucks and the helicopters and all the protestors holding up paperboard signs that read *Stop the Flights*. His wife had called in the middle of the broadcast and asked what she was supposed to say to people asking where he was.

"I'm getting calls from everyone," she said. "What do I tell them?"

"Nothing. Tell them you don't know what's going on."

Henry felt they'd done the right thing. He and

Edminster, the med crew, they'd helped out a man who risked his life to save strangers, and the least they could do was return the favor. Quietly, though. There was no need for everyone to know who was doing it, not when they were getting this mad. He told himself the anonymity was to protect his son, who was in eighth grade and hadn't asked for any of the trouble his dad's job might bring down on him, but really it was for him too. Especially right now.

"Why are they bringing them here?!"

Nods all around the riverfront bar. The television, like every television, was tuned to the news and the news was the Ebola flights. Everyone around Henry was angry.

"They shouldn't be doing it! They shouldn't be here!"

Henry sat on his stool, cheeseburger stalled out halfway to his mouth.

"I'd like to know who's doing it, I'll tell you that."

Hiteshew tried not to look, but he was the only one not yelling and it was starting to show. So to hell with it, he'd join in.

"Yeah!" He shook his burger in mock outrage. "They shouldn't be doing that! What are they thinking?"

"Yeah!"

He motioned to the bartender. "Can I get another round over here?"

60

Darrin Benton was moving slowly that morning. He left Wendy's house and drove the forty minutes up to Cartersville, showered, and then met his mother at church. They sat together in the back row. Neither of them saying anything really, just being there. Together. Afterward his sister called and they talked a while. A friend texted and when he told her that yes, he was going on this second flight, she got worried, which came over like anger and after a few exchanges he cut it off saying, "Look I got a lot going on right now." Darrin's parents lived near the airstrip, and for years now every time he had a flight they'd be there to watch him depart, parked at the end of the runway and waving. He was a little embarrassed about it at first, grown man, parents seeing him off to work. But one afternoon he lifted that Learjet right over their heads into a sky bled through with sunset, and the guy sitting next to him in the right seat said, "I wish my parents would do that."

Unlike the first flight, this one would launch with three pilots. Randy Davis and Martin Bell met Darrin at the airfield. Darrin needed to sleep and volunteered to ride third on the way over. Randy was lead pilot, so while he logged their flight plan and put in a fuel order, Darrin and Martin handled the preflight checklist. Darrin was doing his walk-around when he saw Mark Thompson's car speeding toward him. If Mark's not in his office he's probably flying or fishing or at his farm baling hay on a tractor. But when he drives, he drives fast. He screeched to a stop on the tarmac a few feet from Darrin then swung his long legs out of the car. He strolled over and stood there, belt buckle shining in the sun.

"How'd it go?" Big smile. "With Wendy?"

Darrin shook his head. Here he was about to fly halfway around the world to the one place on Earth nobody wanted to be and the guy sending him there hadn't come to wish him luck but to see how his date had gone.

"It was good."

"Yeah?" Mark peacocked around the aircraft for a minute, proud that he'd set up his friend (again), even though Darrin had blown it the first time. "Good. Good. Don't blow it this time."

Then Randy Davis showed up, and a few minutes later the med crew was there. Jonathan and Vance were once again the nurses but this time they were paired with Dr. Barbara Camp. The internet has made it so anyone with access to the FlightAware service can track an aircraft—and way too many people were trying to track this particular aircraft—so to cloak their whereabouts the flight was given the arbitrary call sign Baxter. Engines on. Baxter reached out to the tower for taxi and clearance. Then down the runway for a blast-off at 5 p.m. on Sunday, August 3, Darrin's parents waving from below and disappearing fast. He slept through the crossing, woke for refuel in the Azores, sat in silence as the plane touched down in Monrovia, and then endured the long van ride to the Kendeja. Lunch, a beer, then off to his cabana at 1:30 Monday afternoon. He laid there a minute then drifted off to sleep.

They met in the lobby at eight o'clock that night. Quick bite to eat then into the van and back through the darkened countryside, *War of the Worlds* radio, the eerie stillness of a country on the brink. The empty airport. Darrin did his walk-around while the med crew hung their plastic. Headlights in the distance announced Nancy's arrival and he stood there, it was midnight, watching the slow approach of the white truck. Wendy had asked if he'd be wearing gloves or a mask for this flight, and he'd said no, that he wouldn't ever be close enough to anyone to need them, and he stayed back now. Well off to the side.

Nancy wasn't loaded like Kent. She couldn't walk, couldn't even stand, and here is where the genius of the Gulfstream III came to bear. They opened the cargo door and a belt loader was extended to the aircraft so Nancy could be carried in on a stretcher. The cargo door is the critical peculiarity Dent and Mark had immediately recognized when Bob Tracey called to say the Danish military was selling off its two remaining Gulfstream III aircraft. It's why they'd since committed their staff to the fraught process of creating their own cargo doors—the flexibility required to be prepared for a job you never expected to do. This capability was great for Phoenix in general but less so in this moment for Jonathan, who had to climb onto the belt loader to ride alongside Nancy's cot, holding on to the edge and way too close to either falling off the loader or getting exposed to the virus. A long week, a longer flight, not even home for a day, and now here he was, dangling in the air.

Darrin watched, sweating in the heat. A man walked up. Friendly. Big smile, the kind of smile that explodes onto someone's face, encompasses everything. A contagious sort of joy. He wanted to know about the crew, to thank them, express his concern for their safety, and praise the effort they'd gone through just to get here. It wasn't until after Nancy had been loaded and they were ready to go that Darrin realized the man so friendly and engaging and interested in their well-being was Nancy's husband David.

Any job can sometimes feel like just a job, one more adventure, but here, standing by the fundamental goodness that David Writebol reflected back at him, Darrin was reminded what it was they did and the reason he'd joined up, why he'd quit his job and gone back to school, rearranged and complicated his life, chased off girlfriends, and (just yesterday) maybe even *friend* friends. To give, to help, to sacrifice. To be of service. Years later he'd struggle to express the magnitude of this one small moment and the way he felt.

At 1 a.m. local time they lifted off from Roberts International Airport and flew to Lajes Air Base for the first leg home. Across the Atlantic a phone rang in DC. Dr. William Walters was at his desk and snatched the receiver.

"Is this Dr. Walters?"

"Yes."

"Dr. William Walters?"

It was late and this game was testing his patience. "Yes."

The caller was an official from the Maine Department of Public Health. "We're considering filing felony charges against you for the improper importation of a Category A pathogen into the State of Maine."

In some ways, this was the call Walters had been waiting for since all this started. He couldn't shake the feeling that they only managed to pull off the Kent Brantly mission because it happened so fast. They got away with the first one. This time they got caught.

Walters leaned back in his chair. "O...kay. Well, I'm operating in the scope of my duties as a federal employee so I'm not sure where that's gonna go." Silence over the line. Then, "Why don't we get to what you're so mad about."

Maine was mad about a lot of things, including that they couldn't do anything to stop the flights because nobody involved in them was answerable to the state. The federal government and its agents—namely Nadeau and Walters—had gone over their heads and it made them feel impotent, and they didn't like it. And they sure as hell didn't want any more flights. These were not what Walters considered legitimate concerns.

"So, guess what? In three hours, there'll be a Gulfstream III landing on the federal ramp in Bangor. I'm sorry you got left out of the communications but you now have all of the information. Is there anything else I can help you with?"

It was the last word from Maine. On the afternoon of Monday, August 4, an aircraft operating under call sign Baxter arrived at Bangor International without incident. If state officials had ever been serious about charging Walters, he'd very quickly made them unserious about it. Nor did they try to interfere with the landing. The only thing awaiting Darrin as he touched down was a text from Wendy asking if he'd like to go with her the following week on a fishing trip to Alaska. Darrin was tired and whiplashed from the roller coaster he'd been on since Friday, hungry because Randy Davis had stepped on the pizzas somewhere off the coast of Liberia, which left them without food for the Atlantic crossing. Now he was buzzing.

Two days ago he thought this relationship was over. But then came their date. And now this. He stopped a moment to consider his response. The last time she showed interest in him he got so excited and moved so quickly that he scared her off and blew the whole thing; this time, despite the night they'd spent together, he'd undersell it. But how do you undersell that you're halfway in love and wouldn't miss that trip, this chance, for anything short of the end of the world, which weirdly, kind of, is exactly what had brought them back together. There *is* no way and anyhow that's not Darrin's style, he's a what-you-see-is-what-you-get kind of guy, so he shot back a fast and excited "Yes, yeah, of course, would love to." Then turned off his phone and settled into his seat. As the aircraft taxied to the customs ramp, he had one overwhelming thought in his head—he had his dream job, his dream girl, and with this sudden and inexplicable turn of events he was maybe, probably, the luckiest person of all time.

61

Whatever Ebola had done for Darrin Benton's love life it had the opposite effect on Gail Stalling's. Online dating had helped bridge the gap between the opportunity to meet someone new and all the time she spent at work. She'd created a profile, started meeting guys, and going on dates. Things in that regard were looking up. Until the day she became famous. The day Kent landed, the day news helicopters and some random weirdo on the highway aimed cameras at her as she made the twenty-five mile drive from Dobbins to Emory with the most famous patient on Earth in the back of her ambulance. She was filmed and photographed, and those images, along with her name, were all over the television and by morning all over the front pages of newspapers around the country. One of the bonuses to online dating is when you match with someone you can immediately look them up, see beyond the profile to who it is you're talking to, and that afternoon if you googled Gail Stallings, about the only thing that'd pop up is the word Ebola. Guys must've been looking her up, because her profile went instantly silent. Matches ceased, messages went unread or un-responded to, and dates were cancelled. She was the Ebola woman.

Which, whatever. John Arevalo, her partner, laughed at her. And in a way it was good, because it gave them something to talk about while waiting for the second plane to arrive and suiting up to once again transport an Ebola patient. They were aware this time would be different. The media was less ravenous this go-round, but their patient was also less stable. In Liberia it'd been Kent teetering on the edge but now, two days later, the ground beneath Nancy Writebol had begun to shift. They knew she couldn't walk and what little had been transmitted to them suggested her potassium was dangerously low. Gail knew that Nancy's heart rhythm was going to be a problem—one of those wildly concerning arrythmias that scared even Ribner—and with it everything else would be skittering toward the edge of trouble. A patient like that, with critical lab levels and scary symptoms to match, was liable to go into cardiac arrest at any time.

Cardiac arrest is a funny term, too often misused, that represents a simple but horrifying truth. Your heart has recently stopped beating and now you're mostly dead. *Mostly* because cardiac arrest is a medical term, which means for it to apply to you someone with medical experience was probably there to name what happened, and in turn that means there's a chance, dimming by the second, that it can be reversed with medical intervention. You're dead but with a chance for a do-over. This is where CPR comes in. CPR is a brutal process. It's also gross. Liquids normally on the inside like vomit and blood and bile have a funny way of shooting out when you're pumping air down someone's throat and pounding on their chest. It's why the protocols Gail and John usually operated under stated, unequivocally, that if someone with a disease like Ebola goes into cardiac arrest you don't even try to save them. It's the opposite of everything a medic is trained, equipped, and deployed to do. Then again, rule number one in EMS is *get home safe*, and stirring up the viral insides of a patient teeming with Ebola is a great way to ensure that rule number one *won't* happen.

But normal protocols for treating cardiac arrest with infectious patients went out the window with Kent and Nancy. The entire world was watching. How would it look if after all that had gone into getting them here, the transport agency had simply let one of them die? No amount of explaining would do; no one would understand or even care to hear their reasons. Forget the dangers; forget that their ambulance didn't carry the amount of IV potassium needed to undo the thing that had killed them in the first place. Forget the risk; forget everything—all the world would see is that they had sat and watched as someone died. So they were told the protocol had changed, that if Kent or Nancy went into arrest, they were to work it, same as any other patient. And that fountain of contaminate liable to come shooting out? Try not to get it on you.

If Nancy were to crash while Gail was alone with her in the back, hampered by the suit, visibility all but zero in the hood, it'd be impossible for her to work the arrest. She needed a second pair of hands. She asked Arevalo to ride in the back with her. AJ, their team leader, agreed to drive them to Emory. Gail and Arevalo were standing by when the aircraft landed and they climbed inside. Her first impression of Nancy was that she was incredibly sick. They got her out of the jet by strapping her to a stair chair—picture a kitchen chair with wheels—then lifted her onto the stretcher. Into the ambulance, the doors closed, and then they were moving.

Mainly their job was to sit there, hoping nothing went wrong but waiting for it happen. To be present. Nancy was exhausted and Gail Stallings just sat on the bench seat and talked to her. Held her hand. Carried her home.

62

The Gulfstream III returned to Cartersville at 2:15 p.m. on Tuesday, August 5, taxied down the runway, shed its crew, and then limped to the far hangar where it sat under armed guard. The medical crew, exhausted beyond measure, climbed back into Tyvek suits to decontaminate the ABCS tent with the chemicals provided them by the CDC, whose experts once again came to supervise but not participate. After decon, Tawn Heater climbed inside, untied the tent's hundreds of fasteners, and then removed, packaged, and sent the ABCS off for incineration. Dent was five hundred yards away in his office. They'd done it. Less than a week and a half from that first phone call from Walters—*my God, Beech Mountain was a lifetime ago*. From a cold start Phoenix Air had spun-up a dizzyingly complicated mission and, what's more, pulled it off. Two desperate people had been brought home. Success.

But there was no elation. The operational part of

the mission was over. Now only the aftermath loomed. Like waking up the morning after a great party, when your eyes first open to the light of a new day and you wonder but don't yet know if there will be a hangover. Dent had his suspicions. They were careful. But how careful was enough? And what about the ABCS—what's the real-world threshold on *thoroughly tested* or *government approved*? It'd been exciting and disorienting, a whirlwind, but the chaos was gone and in its place remained the question of whether or not somebody was going to get sick. Dent was waiting for the other shoe to drop.

Unless someone had a known exposure there'd be no mandatory quarantine period. Through a deal worked out with the Georgia Department of Public Health everyone involved would check their temperature twice a day and report the data and their overall condition to state health officials. Anyone who showed a fever would go immediately to Emory but otherwise they could remain home. It was simple but not all that reassuring. When it's your life on the line, there's always some part of you that would prefer an expert's opinion. The pilots and med crews, all the people who'd been around them since their return, might not have been scared but they were realists. They knew the risks of what they'd done and kept a sort of wary eye on each other.

Getting sick was on everyone's mind, even when they weren't talking about it. It was scary times. Dent never set foot on the aircraft, certainly didn't enter the ABCS, and yet he carried an old mercury thermometer in a glass of alcohol and half-a-dozen times a day he'd shake the thermometer, slip it under his tongue, and anxiously count the seconds until he could check it. He did this at work but also at home, where he kept a thermometer on the vanity in his bathroom. There he was, compulsively taking his temperature, checking to see if an exposure by proxy had given him hemorrhagic fever, before slipping into bed next to Pepper. She could've been forgiven for making him sleep in another room, another house even, but in a way all this was an extension of what Phoenix had always done and she trusted him not to do anything stupid. All the same, she kept in her head a silent tally of Dent's temperature chart.

Dent wasn't alone. The air around Phoenix had stagnated into a climate of nervousness. The general public was afraid of them. Employees went home and were shunned by their neighbors. A maintenance guy was kicked out of a carwash when the employees heard where he worked. Dent cleared an entire Caribou Coffee when the barista recognized him from a story broadcast on television the night before and yelled out, "You're the Ebola guy!" Jonathan Jackson got into an argument with the principal of his daughters' school who told him to stay off campus because he was making the other parents nervous. Larry Goolsby, a flight nurse who alongside Vance Ferebee runs Phoenix Air's medical wing, was briefly detained when officials at Hartsfield-Jackson Atlanta International Airport learned he worked with people who'd recently traveled to West Africa. Then Dr. Mike got a phone call from Dent saying that one of the pilots had admitted during a routine doctor's appointment to working at Phoenix Air. He was immediately locked in an empty exam room and now sat awaiting the arrival of the local police. Dent wanted to know if Dr. Mike could call over there and straighten the whole thing out.

Those first days were a roller coaster of emotion, of pride in what they'd done and also the prickly dread of wondering what it might cost. And it was happening as the scrum of reporters grew larger, the demand for an explanation louder. Looming above it all was the prospect of even more flights. Phoenix had proven itself capable of accomplishing an impossible mission—it was only a matter of time before they were called on to do it again.

63

Linda was hit first by an overwhelming sense of relief. That Kent and Nancy were home and maybe even on the path to recovery was for her a rare bright spot in the most difficult two weeks of her life. She was happy, the whole staff was happy, but their evacuations only highlighted the uncertain fate of the thinning band of volunteers left behind. Any elation they felt at the rescue of their colleagues almost immediately was replaced by the deadening reality that they were hours from being completely overrun. Something had shifted in the country; the virus had taken on a frightening velocity. A surge of patients began flooding in, and no one was coming to help. The medical staff hadn't gotten reinforcements since Kent's diagnosis and after accounting for everyone who'd either rotated out or been evacuated, the number of medical providers working ELWA's Ebola Treatment Center—the only facility of its kind in Monrovia—was four. Four volunteers providing care in a city of one million people.

And those people were getting angry. Among the stubborn legacies of Liberia's civil war were all of its child soldiers. They were older now but still dangerous, still out there. It gave the country a simmering air of danger that Linda could feel. The ELWA hospital compound had a wall around it and a security team but there was a growing crowd just beyond the gates. Some of them had machetes and they wanted to come in, wanted to know what was happening inside. Fear had birthed rumors, and the rumor was that foreign workers were experimenting on patients. Violence seemed a very real possibility. The Ministry of Health had already been burned to the ground. Doctors had been attacked. With her country on the verge of collapse, Liberia's president declared a state of emergency.

Linda was emotionally and physically spent. The previous month had taken an enormous psychological toll on the staff too; they looked shell-shocked. And their role was only growing. A new and much larger treatment center that could hold dozens of patients was nearly complete and, once opened, would need an equally large and energized medical staff to run it. That staff simply did not exist. They reached out to MSF, who agreed to come in and assume control of the new treatment center. No longer in charge but still in the firing line, the leadership of Samaritan's Purse called a meeting to decide whether or not they could go on.

It didn't take long. Shortly after Nancy arrived back home in the US, the organization made the decision to pull their people out of Liberia.

When word arrived of the staff's imminent departure, Linda felt all the stress and fear and anxiety that'd been twisting up inside of her snap and uncoil. It was over and she had nothing left to give. The staff left together on Air France, the only commercial airline to even consider allowing them passage. Their flight to Paris was otherwise empty and from her seat in coach Linda watched as Liberia slipped away beneath her.

64

It wasn't long, a few days at the most, before Dent realized that with Ebola there would be no end. The epidemic was uncontained; the numbers of dead and infected in Guinea, Sierra Leone, and Liberia were rapidly growing. Western governments might still be in denial, but the world's leading epidemiologists began heading to West Africa in ever-increasing numbers. All of them would be in danger and some would come down with fevers that would initially be attributed to exhaustion and then misdiagnosed as malaria before finally the skin would blotch and the eyes would bleed and then the diarrhea and the vomiting and the sweating would confirm the worst. And then Dent's phone would ring. The world would once again turn to Cartersville, and it would continue as long as the outbreak continued, as long as people were dying. But Phoenix had only one modified aircraft, in essence a single ABCS. So from setup to wheels up, to landing in West Africa, crew rest, the flight home, decon, and setting back up again, it was a three-day turnaround for just one mission. And that's if everything went right, if the thousand things that could go wrong *didn't* go wrong. There weren't enough resources, meaning that eventually they'd be put in the horrible position of having to decide where to use them. One day soon the French, for instance, would have a doctor near death, but so would the Italians or the South Africans, maybe, the English, the Indians. And Phoenix would have to make the call on who they rescued. Dent Thompson would have to decide who lived and who died.

Phoenix prided itself on being a lifeboat for the medical community, saving the saviors. They occupied a privileged position but were now coming to grips with what it meant to be the only ones there. The anxiety that had long served as Dent's survival mechanism kicked in. He called an emergency meeting of Phoenix Air's small circle of leadership and laid out the likelihood of their growing role and its *Sophie's Choice* inevitability.

"That happens," he said, "we won't be credited for saving a life. We'll only be blamed for letting someone die."

There were other concerns. The ABCS could technically be considered a medical device, one that had approvals from the government's top engineers and scientists but not from the FDA or the American Medical

Association. What would happen, he asked, if in the use of this unapproved medical device someone died? Could the company be held liable? Could its doctors? Could someone sue them (surely they would), and if that happened where would it leave Phoenix? Even if they won, the whole thing would be devastating. It was a somber counterpoint to the whirlwind week they'd just survived, but they were on the forefront of a world-shaking event and this felt like a necessary reassessment of where they stood.

Dent looked around. "We gotta stop." Heads nodding. "Between the liability and the limited resources and more people looking at us to use them, we can't go on."

It was a reasonable conclusion, something most companies would've arrived at way back in the beginning, during that first phone call. But *no* isn't really part of Phoenix's corporate culture. They're the company that clung to life and slowly grew by transporting the things—dynamite, warheads, smallpox, suitcase nukes—nobody else wanted to touch. This was just an extension of that, albeit an insane one, and together they agreed on a way forward. That afternoon Dent called the CDC and the State Department and he told them each the same thing. If the US government wanted them to continue carrying out Ebola rescue missions, then the government needed to take full control of those missions.

"We're not doing any more Ebola flights," he said. "Not unless we have a partner to take us to the dance."

He hung up. He waited. The CDC called back to say they were holding meetings to determine what a contract might look like. That sounded to Dent like a long process, and he went to bed that night figuring he'd bought himself a little time, who knows, maybe a lot of time—he hadn't yet heard from the State Department and didn't know what their response would be. He drove to work the next morning and had barely settled in when Walters came bursting through the door. He had a federal contract officer with him, and two hours later Dent was signing an emergency deal to keep going. Phoenix Air was now the official Ebola airline of the US Department of State.

PART FOUR

65

DEEP IN THE HIMALAYAS
MARCH 13, 2020

At a community hospital outside of Paro, Bhutan, a seventy-six-year-old doctor lay dying. A ventilator breathed for him. He was unconscious beneath a tangled collection of tubes and wires. Healthcare workers entered his room in biohazard suits and carefully, because even the air around him was contagious, prepared him for transport. Fifty miles away a Gulfstream III aircraft—gunmetal gray, modified with a cargo door, and outfitted with an ABCS—sliced through the air a hundred feet off the Paro Chhu River. Overhead the advance guard of a predicted snowstorm pressed in on a bank of gray clouds. The weather would not hold; snow was coming. Because of the steep, mountainous topography, radar does not work in the Paro Valley. The pilot flew by sight, without a navigation system, hands on the stick as he followed the meandering course of a Himalayan river north into the heart of Bhutan. Eighteen-thousand-foot peaks towered from all sides, roof of the world, the jet absolutely streaking along just to keep its fingertip hold on the thin air. A final bend in the river, a harrowing 45-degree turn, and at last Paro International, one of the world's most dangerous airports, appeared in the windscreen—a tiny runway at the bottom of a Himalayan bowl. Corkscrew in, moving fast, stopping faster, veer off course even a little and the jet plows into the houses lining either side. The pilot banked and held course. The onboard systems screamed their warning: *Terrain ahead, pull up, pull up!*

It was March 13, 2020. A Friday. The last six years had been a blur.

The agreement Dent signed with Walters that day in August 2014 was a six-month emergency contract that essentially handed to the State Department control of the modified Gulfstream III aircraft, its flight crew, the medical team, the ABCS, and all the equipment necessary to transport a patient in full isolation. Ebola isn't traditionally something you'd look on as a growth opportunity, but with the stroke of a pen Phoenix Air sprang from its role as lifeline to a single NGO and became a lifeline for the entire world. Walters already had another mission planned, with more on the way, and as Dent walked back to his office that afternoon in 2014 the overriding thought was, *How big will this get?*

Kent Brantly was certain when he and Nancy Writebol were diagnosed with Ebola at the ELWA hospital in late July that one of them would die. Maybe both. The case mortality rate for Zaire Ebola during the 2014 West Africa outbreak was staggering. For weeks Kent lived in a fog, his existence shrunk to a single mattress, scared and slowly dying, haunted by the guilt that Nancy had gotten sick on his watch. Then, on August 18, the universe shifted. For the first time since her diagnosis and almost two weeks after arriving at Emory, consecutive blood tests found no traces of the virus in Nancy's body. She was transferred out of the Serious Communicable Disease Unit. Nancy Writebol, who arrived in the US later than Kent and much sicker, had healed first. Two days later, almost exactly a month after his symptoms began, Kent got the same news. He was released to a step-down unit and then, finally, back into the world.

Emory held a press conference the day Kent walked out. The doctor who contracted Ebola, whose name and face had flashed all over the world, whose groundbreaking rescue mission was still being debated, finally spoke. He stood for six and a half minutes before the international press that'd been living outside Emory University Hospital. He thanked the doctors at Emory, his coworkers in Liberia, his family and friends, God, and called the day miraculous. But there was work to be done and he planned to use his newfound celebrity to shake the world's consciousness.

He was named, along with other Ebola doctors, *Time* magazine's Person of the Year. He appeared on *The Today Show*. He flew to Washington, DC, and met with President Barack Obama in the Oval Office. He spoke before a House subcommittee, begged them to step in and provide the aid West Africa so desperately needed. Since the preceding spring when an Ebola outbreak was first declared, the international community, which hadn't yet recognized the full scale of the problem, had stood by and allowed two relief agencies to provide all the care for victims of an epidemic that had spread out across an entire region of Africa. Those agencies were not nearly enough and the virus was now uncontained and out of control.

"The response to date has remained sluggish," Kent said. "We cannot fool ourselves into thinking that the vast moat of the Atlantic Ocean will protect us."

That the virus could extend beyond, far beyond, the borders of the three countries it'd overtaken seemed obvious and in fact had already happened. On July 20, 2014, a Liberian-born American named Patrick Sawyer boarded a commercial flight out of Monrovia for Lagos, Nigeria. He felt fine boarding the plane but arrived in Lagos near death. He was weak and vomiting. He collapsed, was rushed to First Consultants Medical Centre, and there he tested positive for Ebola. A quick investigation led back to Sawyer's sister, now dead. He'd been her caretaker before leaving Liberia on an airliner. After her death, he boarded a plane, had a brief layover in Togo, and now was in Nigeria. A short itinerary, three countries, hundreds of passengers all headed in different directions. Sawyer himself had landed in a teeming city of twenty-one million people.

As he spiraled toward death, public health officials in Nigeria scrambled to stop the virus. They traced contacts and quarantined passengers, flights were cancelled, entire airlines pulled out of Freetown in Sierra Leone, and Monrovia in Liberia. Nigeria in 2012 had instituted a polio eradication program and doctors used that same framework now to contain Ebola. The virus spread to only twenty people, killing eight, including several healthcare workers. Sawyer died on July 25, the first American killed by the virus. He was also, briefly, the vector that experts had always feared. This was the inevitability that made Dr. Anthony Fauci, the director of the National Institute of Allergy and Infectious Diseases, believe we were staring into the abyss. And this was the very reasoning CDC Director Tom Friedan had given as justification for flying Kent and Nancy to the US—if you don't protect the people going to fight an outbreak, they stop going; and if they stop going, the outbreak spreads and once it starts to spread it'll never stop.

The message at last was received. President Obama deployed four thousand US troops to Liberia. Organizations such as USAID spun up operations. Other governments and more experts followed. The fight was on to stop Ebola, and in the midst of all this activity was a small company with a strange reputation that happened to have the one thing nobody else had. If Dent's question was *How big could this get?*, then the answer was *very big*.

66

The first two Ebola flights were essentially private transactions, and they happened so fast that Walters could more or less wave a wand and make rules go away. Starting with the third, everything changed. With everyone watching and the government in charge, everything had to be done by the rules. And since nearly every aspect of these transports broke the rules, the rules would have to change. A whole raft of federal regulations concerning aircraft, flight crews, and the transportation of hazardous material had to be rewritten and changed into law. They needed a permanent place to land, something closer and easier to monitor than Bangor International. The government chose Dulles, just across the Potomac from DC, and secured a place hidden in the back and far from everyone else. They rewrote laws about mandatory quarantines and crew rest and even the laws regulating what could be transported over US highways so that used biocontainment systems could be hermetically sealed and transported north on I-75 from Hartsfield-Jackson International Airport in Atlanta to Cartersville.

And they finally got a long-term plan for decontamination when Dent was introduced to Clay Wardlaw, who ran a medical-grade decon business. Clay watched Dr. Mike decontaminate the Gray Bird after the third flight, then walked into Dent's office.

Clay shook his head. "This ain't good."

He started explaining his own process for decon, describing how the vaporized hydrogen peroxide he used is classified as jet fuel and corrosive enough to pit metal. By this point Dent was already dialing Walters, who listened for a minute and said, "Put this guy under contract right now."

Which he did. And before the ink was dry on that contract the Gray Bird was in the air and on its way back to Monrovia.

67

Linda Mobula had returned home to a life she didn't know. Before Liberia she'd rented an apartment in Silver Springs, Maryland, but hadn't lived in it, and now she had a new job with USAID but hadn't started there. Coming home was like stepping into some other version of herself, the wrong version, and what she wanted was to be back in Liberia.

Her new job at USAID didn't start until September, which meant she had nothing but time to sit around and think. And all she could think about was the outbreak. It weighed heavily on her and never left, even though she had. That's what bothered her the most. That she'd gone there, as she'd gone to other disasters, to see it through, and when everything came apart she got on an airplane and escaped. By now the new Ebola Treatment Center was open, and instead of suiting up for a shift, she was here, watching the outbreak on television.

Mountains were moved to evacuate Kent and

Nancy, and once they were home she got out of Liberia too. These things gave her a sense of relief and accomplishment but left her conflicted because no such rescue awaited Liberians. Consider Barbara Bono, a Liberian ER nurse who worked alongside Linda at ELWA. Barbara was helping a patient back to bed when he lost his balance and grabbed her arm. Sunk his fingernails through the skin. Within days she had a fever and got tested and that test came back positive for Ebola. From provider to patient in an instant, brought into the ETC watching people die all around her, watching her colleagues struggle to keep up, thinking of her two young daughters and how they'd be left all alone if she died. Barbara spent fourteen days in the ETC and then emerged as if from another world, cured, one of the miracles, a testament to the care and passion of the staff at ELWA but also a reminder that the care for locals was different than it was for Westerners.

That fact nagged at her, contributed to the voices of doubt and frustration that echoed in her head late at night. The only way to quiet them was to go back.

68

With the world suddenly stampeding into West Africa, the number of missions Phoenix flew dramatically increased. Their patients were no longer just Americans. They were doctors and nurses from all over the world. Most had been working in West Africa for an NGO when they were exposed. Nearly all were symptomatic. Two of them died. Dr. Mike had an exposure when the sleeve of his Tyvek suit lifted up as he was moving a patient; one of the medics was doused from head to toe in bloody vomit; Jonathan had to run into the ABCS mid-flight when a confused and agitated patient tried to break out. Darrin Benton was ready to take off from Sierra Leone with an Ebola patient when his left engine wouldn't start. He tried to fix it, couldn't, and so he called Rickey Smith. It was 2 a.m. on the East Coast, but Rickey took the call and listened to the problem and then walked him through the fix, which was a lot of *blow on this, turn off that, flip these switches*. Darrin asked if anything could go wrong, and Rickey, back home lying in bed, said, "Yeah, but you're down anyway. Might as well try."

Henry Hiteshew touched down in France one night and was met on the runway by a colonel who drew his pistol, pointed it at the windshield, and yelled, "Stay on the plane!" Brian Edminster was with him on that flight, though he remembers it happening in Germany. The fact that neither of the pilots is clear on where exactly they were when a high-ranking member of a foreign military pointed a gun at their heads suggests just how crazy a time it was.

The epidemic of 2014–2016 was the largest Ebola outbreak since the virus was discovered in 1976 and the first to occur in a major urban area. By the time it was officially declared over in June 2016, nearly thirty thousand people had become infected and over eleven thousand had died. And somehow—call it a lack of preparation or imagination or courage, perhaps—Phoenix Air was the only company flying medevac missions. Their pilots transported blood samples, specialized equipment, and medications; Dr. Mike volunteered to take part in a medical trial for an Ebola vaccine developed in conjunction with Emory University Hospital where Bruce Ribner, armed with a bevy of new data, shared what he'd learned with his counterparts in West Africa and helped to significantly reduce mortality rates there. Phoenix eventually modified a second Gulfstream III, and in total flew more than forty missions, bringing doctors of various nationalities to definitive care facilities around the world. Their last Ebola evacuation flight took off out of Sierra Leone on April 10, 2015.

A postmortem on the United States' Ebola response revealed a significant and recurring problem—a lack of capacity. The US could handle a small problem, a one-off, but nothing larger. Not easily. Specifically, there weren't enough specialized facilities to receive patients and definitely not enough aircraft to bring them there. Some of this was the product of an almost willful refusal to prepare. Ribner's lab within the Serious Communicable Disease Unit at Emory had been shut down, as had the Grady EMS Special Operations Team. Only a handful of hospitals could safely handle patients with highly infectious diseases, and no one but Phoenix Air was in a position to move them. Something had to change. Ribner began speaking at conferences and consulting for hospitals in an effort to spread the knowledge contained inside his Serious Communicable Disease Unit. Slowly, one bed at a time, hospital capacity increased. But transportation remained an issue. The ABCS, as innovative as it was, could only move one patient at a time. It was too small. This was the realization that birthed the Containerized Biocontainment System (CBCS). The Paul G. Allen Family Foundation donated $5 million to the problem. The technology and science firm MRIGlobal designed a large-scale mobile isolation unit capable of transporting multiple patients at once. The CBCS, made to fit a 747, revolutionized the treatment and transportation of patients with highly infectious diseases but, like the ABCS before it, by the time the units were ready for use the immediate threat was over. The half-dozen CBCS units manufactured were left in hangars, waiting for the next outbreak.

69

Rumors first arose in the fall of 2019 of a strange new virus in Wuhan, China. As cases, and then deaths, spiked, the State Department began evacuating Americans. Two CBCS units were loaded into a pair of government 747s to evacuate the US diplomatic corps. This was followed soon after by the evacuation of Americans living in the area for business. Inside the containers, treating patients and running the units, were Phoenix Air medical and maintenance staff. As COVID-19 spread, five rescues were flown out of Wuhan—1,100 people, all treated by Phoenix medics. Next came the *Diamond Princess*, a cruise ship in Yokohama, Japan. It was February 2020, COVID-19 was running wild on the boat, and Phoenix evacuated 328 Americans. Together these two missions in China and Japan constituted the largest evacuation of civilians in US history. They did it again in March, evacuating 140 foreign nationals from the *Grand Princess* cruise ship, which at the time was docked in Oakland, California.

In 2020 alone, on both the CBCS and, occasionally the ABCS, Phoenix took part in over 1,000 rescue flights into 136 countries, delivering 178,000 pounds of medical cargo and supplies and repatriating more than 100,000 Americans. Their engineers developed freezers large enough to hold a significant amount of supplies, but safe and light enough to be transported by aircraft. Then, in the summer of 2021, they helped deliver COVID-19 vaccines to US embassies across the world. Much of this was run through the State Department where Walters, who viewed Ebola as a dry run for what was unfolding in 2020, aggressively scheduled rescue missions on the simple theory that people want to die at home; either you bring them back safely or they'll find a way on their own.

It was with this in mind that he called Phoenix on March 10, 2020. A seventy-six-year-old American doctor in Bhutan had been diagnosed with COVID-19, part of that first wave of patients, the wave that confounded doctors. The wave that wound up on ventilators. That died in alarming numbers. Efforts were underway to evacuate him from Bhutan to an ICU in Baltimore. It was a nearly eight-thousand-mile flight with massive logistical challenges. He was incredibly sick and getting sicker and the mission needed to happen now; a plane would have to land at Paro International, an airport so difficult to reach—radar didn't work, the weather was notoriously bad, the elevation was dizzying, the runway a matchstick—that flights weren't allowed in unless they had a locally trained navigator to lead the way. And there was also the fact that airports around the world were closing as COVID-19 spread. All this plus the heavy snow that was predicted for Friday evening. Any delays and the mission would be off. Permanently.

Phoenix's closest ABCS-equipped Gulfstream III was stationed in Kenya. The nearest pilot, Cheyenne Foote, coming off a long trip and at the Nairobi airport, was about to fly home. When he got the call, he went back to the check-in counter, grabbed his bag back from the carousel, and headed to the FBO where the aircraft was waiting. Whether they'd have an open airport to leave from was very much in question.

But the airports did stay open, the weather held, and on Thursday one of the dozen or so navigators certified to fly into Paro International was located in the Indian city of Kolkata. Cheyenne and copilot Greg McPherson took off from Nairobi, grabbed the navigator in Kolkata, and then flew into Bhutan. After a few hours, the plane began its descent into the Paro Valley and, with Cheyenne flying by hand, the navigator told him to drop down low over the river and follow its contours through the mountains. Cheyenne was one of Phoenix's most experienced pilots, but this was difficult flying. When the airport finally came into view the navigator pointed toward a row of buildings crowding the airstrip. "Aim at that green roof there."

A steep drop into a short runway, screaming in over the buildings, gear down, full flaps, spoilers deployed, brakes, thrust reversers, seventy-thousand pounds of jet-propelled metal, and the end of the runway coming up fast. But he did it. The aircraft screeched to a halt. They were stopped but would quickly have to move. The storm was coming fast, the afternoon winds had already begun picking up. The med crew threw on PPEs, scrambled out, and loaded the patient through the cargo door. Once the ventilator and pumps and monitors keeping him alive were all checked and adjusted, the cargo door swung shut and the aircraft turned its nose toward the runway. The navigator was required to fly in but not out and he wanted to stay, so Cheyenne and McPherson would have to navigate the Himalayas by memory. The Gray Bird's two Rolls-Royce jet engines spun up as the aircraft gained speed and lifted off, just barely, at the end of the runway. Thirty hours later they touched down in Baltimore. The patient, whose rescue the US Secretary of State Michael Pompeo called "the most complex medical evacuation in history," would make a full recovery. After dropping him off, the Gray Bird, looking like a clown car and packed tight with a half-dozen pilots, two nurses, and a medic—all of them exhausted and unshowered, definitely hungry, and most likely ready for a beer—flew the final leg home on a cloud of shit talk and jet fuel and more than just a little pride.

70

Throughout the Ebola epidemic Phoenix Air remained the only hope of rescue for the world's medical experts. That capacity expanded during the COVID-19 pandemic to include not only government experts, but ordinary citizens who fell sick far from home. By then Dr. Mike had retired and Doug Olson took over as medical director. Which was fitting. Doug had served as doctor on the first flight in July 2014 and was there at the end, for the last flight, the following year. Doug flew eleven Ebola missions, and when it was over he stayed quiet and tried to move on with his life. He was after all the doctor who'd spent years practicing medicine in dangerous places; the guy who had chased danger across the world and described himself as having an abnormally low response to stress. He admitted his role in the missions only when he had to. He wanted to do his job and then, when it was over, melt back into the world like it'd never happened.

And he did. Until the day he heard that Kent and

Amber Brantly had written a book about their experience and would be in Atlanta for an event. He wasn't sure what he'd say but he wanted to go, just to see the man whose life he'd helped save. It was evening. Doug walked into the venue, slipped in line, and waited his turn. When Doug got to the front he paused. It'd been a while since that flight and they'd both been through so much. Kent hadn't seen anything but Doug's eyes, Amber had never seen him at all. They wouldn't recognize him, wouldn't know him. What was he doing here? Doug stepped forward. Looked down at Kent.

"I don't know if you know who I am—"

That's as far as he got. Kent hadn't seen Doug's face and didn't know his name but he recognized his voice. How could he not? During the most difficult time of Kent's life Doug had been there to bring him home. For six months, Doug and his coworkers at Phoenix Air had put themselves at tremendous risk, they'd endured long days and endless flights, they'd walked into a hot zone protected by nothing but the PPE they'd bought at Home Depot, faced the anger of a scared country, were ostracized by their neighbors, and hounded by the media. There were exposures and quarantines and even fevers, but they brought people home. Somehow they brought people home. Doug understood at the time that what they were doing was historic, but the bigger question had always been present: Was it right?

Many people at the time thought it was a bad idea, some still did. Were the lives they saved worth the risk?

The last time he saw Kent, Doug wasn't sure that he'd survive. Now, at the sound of his voice, Kent jumped up. He had lived and was here now, throwing his arms around Doug, in no small part because Doug was the type of American who believed that being a small part of a greater whole required the willingness to serve others, even at risk to yourself. Doug had done that, he'd played his part, and his reward was this—Kent's understanding that when he was dying and needed help, someone came for him.

ACKNOWLEDGMENTS

This book wouldn't have been possible without the energy and enthusiasm—the will-it-into-life insistence—of Dent Thompson. I first met Dent seven years ago, another former ambulance man who left the streets but found they never left him. In the years since, scarcely has a month gone by when Dent hasn't reached out with the kind of wild Phoenix Air story that ends, as his Southern drawl devolves into a squeal, with him crowing, *You can't make this shit up*. Dent is a P. T. Barnum for our age. When I moved with my family to Atlanta, he invited me out to Cartersville. There I was given the tour normally reserved for members of the State Department and the Department of Defense, a whirlwind of facts and figures and technology, of mildly confused machinists, mechanics, engineers, pilots, and doctors pulled from their work and told to explain to me exactly what it is they do and how. It was during that tour, but before lunch (it really is all about lunch at Phoenix) that I saw the ABCS and heard about Ebola and realized I was standing in the middle of an incredible story. That this was almost certainly Dent's intention from the start didn't occur to me until much later. Well played, Dent.

Mark Thompson—google him, what you'll find is almost too incredible to believe—has lived an extraordinary life. That he was willing to share so much of it with me, to open the doors of the company he created so I could wander freely and collect its stories, speaks to an openness and generosity rarely found. I remain, like so many others, an indebted admirer.

I want to extend a thank you to everyone at Phoenix. Their sense of purpose and service, their ability to laugh while chaos and danger and impossibility swirl around them, is inspiring. I especially want to thank Jonathan, Vance, Doug, Chris, Tobin, and Tawn for their willingness, repeatedly, to field my questions.

Special thanks to Dr. Mike, whose selflessness and humanity inspired a whole new chapter in my own life; to Darrin and Wendy, who fell in love amidst disaster but did not eat the buttermilk pie; and to Dr. Linda Mobula, whose skill, compassion, and courage have carried her into the darkest moments of our time and who has emerged, repeatedly and improbably, with her humor and grace intact.

On an early June morning in the summer of 2023, my phone rang as I stood in the middle of the Mojave Desert. It was my editor, Brant Rumble. The call started with him rattling off all the things he loved about my latest proposal and ended with an offer to publish the book. It's the phone call every writer dreams about. As always, it never would've happened without Alice, my champion. Thank you.

Above all, my ultimate thanks goes to Pepe, who knows how much goes work into every word and who, having read nothing more than the opening of the first draft, turned to me and said, "OK, I'm in."

www.ingramcontent.com/pod-product-compliance
Lightning Source LLC
LaVergne TN
LVHW031536060526
838200LV00056B/4515